Ab Workout

How to Build Athletic and Powerful Abs

(Best Abs Workout for Core Abs Strength, Building Abdominal Muscles, Six-packs, and Flat Stomach)

Marvin Smith

Published By **Oliver Leish**

Marvin Smith

Ab Workout: How to Build Athletic and Powerful Abs (Best Abs Workout for Core Abs Strength, Building Abdominal Muscles, Six-packs, and Flat Stomach)

ISBN   978-1-77485-925-4

Legal & Disclaimer

TABLE OF CONTENTS

Introduction

Are you curious about foraging and how to harvest and cook edible wild plants? Do you want to learn to identify these plants and learn their benefits, and how to grow them yourself? This book aims to introduce you to the fascinating world of foraging in the wild and how to harvest edible wild plants.

A recent trend has emerged in society; more and more people feel an increasing need to reconnect with nature and take a break from modern-day technology. Conscious of the ecological delicacy of the world, they are trying to find more sustainable food sources. Many have already shifted to plant-based diets, and their numbers are swelling, and there's an increasing demand for organic plant sources to diversify daily meals. If you're already incorporating many fruits and vegetables into your diet, you're probably getting bored with the lack of variety available in the grocery store. You'll want to look for newer ingredients that are healthy, sustainable, and affordable. Organic produce is becoming more widely available, but sometimes it can be quite expensive and limited.

For those reasons, foraging has been gaining popularity in recent years. It's a great way to exercise, breathe some fresh air, and stimulate your innate ability to grow food. In this book, you will learn how to identify different herbs, mushrooms, fruits, nuts, and vegetables in the wild, which you can use in your recipes. You'll be able to understand foraging and learn the tools needed when you're picking plants in the wild. If you're interested in growing wild plants in your backyard, you'll need to learn a few tips and tricks outlined in this book. You'll learn how to plant your seeds, which tools are required, and how to tend to your garden.

Foraging isn't something you'll be doing every day. Depending on where you are, you can find wild plants growing naturally in your garden, on a sidewalk, at a park, or in nearby forests and wild areas. However, some people don't have access to these places and need to take a trip to an area where foraging is allowed. This is why you'll need to learn ways to keep wild plants as fresh as possible. By reading this book, you will find out how to properly preserve and store wild plants, so they last a long time. You'll also need to learn safety rules for storage to ensure the plants don't go bad.

Some wild plants are the same fruits, vegetables, and seeds you find in the grocery store. These plants are easy to include in your recipes because you're used to them. But you may not know how to use other less common wild plants in your recipes. This is why we've included a few recipes in the book to show you how to brighten and spice up your meals using plenty of interesting ingredients found in nature.

Many of these wild plants have amazing medicinal benefits. The great thing about foraging is that you're guaranteed the best quality of plants. You won't find fresher produce that's fertilizer- and pesticide-free. The great thing about wild plants is that they are cultivated by nature. Once you try the fruits and vegetables found in nature, you'll notice they taste heavenly and much better than store-bought plants, even if they were organic. After reading this book, you'll want to get started on foraging for wild plants and using them in your daily recipes.

This book is a comprehensive guide providing you with all the tips you need to successfully forage for edible wild plants. It's important to get acquainted with the types of plants suitable for consumption and learn the poisonous varieties to avoid using them. Let's get started on the world of foraging and how to harvest and cook edible wild plants.

Chapter 1: A Guide to Edible Plants

Food plays a critical role in human socio-cultural and biological existence. Since time immemorial, humans have been sourcing food from the wild, which has helped them develop a knowledge base about edible plants they have since domesticated. Thousands of nutritious and delicious botanicals grow in different places, but other species can also be harmful.

A wide range of plants and their leaves, flowers, seeds, fruits, and underground organs are consumed. Plants provide micronutrients, essential minerals, proteins, and vitamins necessary to our nutritional requirements, and they add quality. This chapter discusses different types of wild edible plants such as herbs, mushrooms, nuts, fruits, and seeds. We also explain the difference between flowers, plants, and weeds.

What Is an Edible Plant?

An edible plant is usually a vegetable - be it green, yellow, orange, purple, red, or a mix of colors, and variety has its own uses and nutrients. We eat different parts of the whole plant in our diets - either roots, leaves, stems, tubers, buds, seeds, flowers, and fruits, raw or cooked. The most common plants are available at our grocery store, either fresh or frozen. However, with the move toward healthier choices, people are adding more and different plants to their diet, and some of these grow wild. But some wild plants can be toxic to humans, so it's wise to be aware of what is safe and what isn't. Being able to tell the difference is a skill. Many things can indicate whether a plant is poisonous, and they include the following:

• Milky sap

• Three leaved foliage

• Pods with beans, bulbs, or seeds

• Fine hairs, thorns, or spines on the stems or leaves

• Stems with almond scent

• Bitter or soapy flavor

• Purple, pink, or black parks on the grain head

If a plant has any of these characteristics, it might be toxic. However, different wild plants are nutrient-rich, although they might have specific features. You need to understand the appropriate methods to use when preparing these foods.

Popular Edible Wild Plants

There are hundreds of edible wild species that grow in different places across the globe. Many plants are associated with the cultures of various tribes or communities, and they can also symbolize many things. The following are some of the common wild edible plants consumed in different areas.

Dandelion

Dandelion is a common weed found in all parts of the world, and it has been a staple food across different cultures. All parts of the plant are edible and can be eaten at every stage of its growth lifecycle. This plant is rich in vitamins A, B, and C, and it also boasts high levels of iron and magnesium. Dandelions belong to the sunflower family and are characterized by their hairless and smooth leaves with toothed edges and yellow flowers.

The other feature of this plant is that it has hollow stems and a wide root system. To harvest this plant, you should pick the leaves when they are tender and most nutritious during the early days of spring and harvest the bright yellow buds before they begin to flower because they quickly develop into seeds.

Asparagus

Asparagus is one of the most popular plants you are most likely to find flourishing in spring, which is the best time to go foraging for food. Asparagus grows abundantly in spring and can easily be found along irrigation ditches and roadsides in loose and sandy soils. This is a perennial plant that produces new growth every year. In the fall, you can identify asparagus plants by their orange and yellow stems and scattered berries under the bushy growth. You can mark the location and harvest the tender green stems when they are ready. The stems should have a white base with a tight, slightly purple crown.

Nettle

Nettle is one of the most nutritious edible wild plants and has a rich mineral flavor. It makes a delicious substitute for kale or spinach. The plants grow approximately three feet, and they have green toothed leaves that grow in the opposite direction. Small hairs also grow on the underside of the leaves, and they can cause sharp stings if you pick them up without gloves. Nettle plants usually grow along riverbeds in partially shady areas.

Nettle leaves are eaten fresh in fresh in salads, especially when you pick them young. When they are still tender, they do not have the stinging qualities which develop as the plat matures. You can also neutralize the stinging by steaming the edible leaves. Boil the leave to use in stir-fries, casseroles, pasta, and pies is another method to prepare the leaves. You can also dry them and keep them in a cool, dry place. Dried nettle leaves make a very good medicinal tea.

Garlic Mustard

Garlic mustard is a common weed found in most parts of North America and Europe. However, many rangers and gardeners revile this plant since it devastates the botanical diversity in many places, and many seeds will not germinate when planted where garlic mustard has previously grown. While the plant is destructive, it is also tasty. Garlic mustard has deep green round leaves with scalloped edges and pronounced veining. You can look for these squat bushy herbs on forest floors during early spring. The plant also sends out long flowering stems with small white four-petal flowers. If you are not certain about your identification of garlic mustard, you can crush a few leaves using your hands, and they will release a garlicky aroma. It can be used as a spice, adding an enticing aroma to your favorite dish.

Elderberry

Elderberries have a musky scent and have been used for making wine for several centuries. They also have a powerful medicinal value are high in flavanols, Vitamin C, and antioxidants. These plants look very similar to the deadly water hemlock, so make sure you can tell the difference between them. Only the berries and flowers are the edible parts and the rest are toxic.

Elderberries grow in moist areas, and the bushes can grow up to 12 feet tall. The stems are woody and brown and have a bark-like appearance near the base of the stem. The leaves are elongated, light green, and have serrated edges that grow in opposite directions. The clusters of white flowers with petals that develop from the light green stems can help you identify the flowering elderberry plants.

You can identify the flowering elderberry plants by the clusters of white flowers with petals that develop from light green stems.

The dark purple berries are visible in summer, forming umbrella-shaped clusters of about 20 fruits. You can use the flowers and berries to make infusions, cordials, wine, and tea, or you can bake them into cakes, cookies, and pies. You should wait until the berries are mature if you want to enjoy their quality taste.

Wild Raspberry

Wild raspberries are one of the most delicious wild fruits and come in different colors. They grow abundantly in wooded areas, and the edible fruits usually emerge during the hot late summer months. Raspberries differ from blackberries in that they have hollow-cored fruits and strong vertical canes with small to medium clustered thorns. You must look for a plant with light-green and spade-shaped leaves that are slender and serrated. Before eating the berries, wash them first, and you can enjoy them raw if you want to get the best nutritional value. You can also add them to your favorite baking recipes for enhanced tartness.

Curled Dock

These plants are found in different parts of the world, especially South and North America, Europe, and Australia. They are characterized by elongated and wavy green leaves that have a slightly sour taste when you eat them raw. Mature plants have tightly clustered flower heads that can change from the usual green to reddish-brown during pollination. They also have long edible reddish stalks, which you should boil first to remove the tough outer layer and then two or three more times, changing the water in between so you get rid of the bitter taste.

While foraging is an amazing way of exploring nature, enriching your diet, and conserving ecosystems, knowing which plants are edible is vital. For instance, curled dock plants are edible, but you may not enjoy them if you don't know how to prepare them. It is a good idea to begin your foraging journey under the guidance of an experienced person who has in-depth knowledge of local plants. If you are in doubt, find better means of testing the plants before consuming them.

Root Vegetables

There are different types of edible underground plants consumed by people in different parts of the globe. Like any other edible plant, root vegetables have high nutritional properties, and they are often identified as tuberous and tape roots. Other non-roots include corms, bulbs, and tubers, although some types consist of hypocotyls and taproot tissues. The term root veggies applies to different plants used for culinary purposes, providing food to people and animals.

Root vegetables are good storage organs that can store large energy volumes in the form of carbohydrates. They also differ from plant to plant in the carbohydrate concentration and nutrient levels, which are made up of sugars, starches, and other forms of carbohydrates. Root veggies high in carbohydrate concentration also provide commercial value since they form staple foods, especially in tropical regions. These foods overshadow most cereals in West Africa, Oceania, and Central Africa, where they are mashed to make foods like fufu. This is a staple diet that is obtained directly from root vegetables.

Many root vegetables can last several months if you store them in root cellars. After harvesting these edible plants, make sure you keep them in a cool, dry place. The harvested crop can last longer if it is free from moisture. The following are examples of root vegetables.

- Konjac

- Taro

- Chinese water chestnut

- Waterlily

- Enset

- Arrowhead or wapatoo

- Malanga, tannia, cocoyam, yautia, and others

- Japanese potato

There are also other rhizome types of edible roots used for different purposes. They include turmeric, ginseng, vanilla lily, rengarenga, canna, lotus root, ginger, galangal, and bulrush.

Yam tubers are other types of edible plants that are added to different dishes. In other cultures, these foods are consumed raw, or they can be cooked. They include the following:

- Tigernut or chufa

- Groundnut or hog potato

- Yams

- Chinese yam

- Sunchoke or Jerusalem artichoke

- Daylily

- Potato

- New Zealand Yam

- Kembili, dazo, and others

- Earthnut pea

- Mashua

Root-like stems are also edible parts of plants, and they can be used as a staple food or added to specific dishes. They include different types of roots with substantial hypocotyls tissue. The following are examples of roots that belong to these categories.

- Arracacha

- Beet and mangelwurzel

- Rutabaga, kohlrabi, and turnip

- Black cumin

- Family Aceraceae

- Daucus carota subsp

- Apium graveolens

- Arctium

- East Asian white radish

- Pastinaca sativa

- Parsley root

- Murnong

- Bush carrot or bush potato

- Black salsify

Other types of edible roots are known as cassava tuberous. These roots are consumed in different forms and can be added to dishes depending on your preferred recipe. The following are examples of cassava roots.

- Native Ginger

- Pignut or earthnut

- Yellow lily yam

- Sweet potato

- Chinese yam, Korean yam, Mountain yam, nagaimo

- Desert yam

- Breadroot, prairie turnip, tipsin

- Cassava or manioc, or yucca

- Yacon

Depending on where you live, different types of edible roots can be found. You can get some of these foods from the bush, while others have since been cultivated for domestic consumption.

Culinary Herbs and Spices

There are several types of culinary herbs and spices specifically used as food or drink additives. Others are used for flavoring and coloring various recipes of food. The following herbal plants are found in different areas and are used for several purposes.

- Allspice

- Cayenne pepper

- Dill herb or weed

- Basil, Holy

- Chili pepper

- Garlic

- Basil, lemon

- Garlic chives

- Borage

- Indonesian bay leaf

- Lavender

- Lesser calamint

- Asafetida

- Cumin

- Shiso

- Alkanna tinctoria
- Licorice
- Indian Bay leaf
- Mbongo spice
- Horseradish
- Para cress
- Celery leaf
- Vanilla
- Chervil
- Oregano
- Galangal, lesser
- Thyme
- Cicely, sweet cicely
- Parsley
- Wild thyme
- Tonka beans
- Galangal, greater
- Lemon ironbark
- Lemongrass

- Basil, Thai

- Perilla

- Boldo

- Peppermint

- Dill seed

- Saffron

- Avens

- Kudum Puli

- Mace

- Blue fenugreek

- Golpar

- Rosemary

- Finger root

- Safflower

- Cinnamon, white

- Locust beans

- Blue melilot

- Lemon verbena

- Annatto

- Jalapeño

- Lime flower

- Celery seed

- Pipicha

- Angelica archangelica

- Ginger

- Pepper

- Tasmanian pepper

- Black onion seed

- Mustard plant

- Rue

- Artemisia

- Quassia

- Epazote

- Wattleseed

- New Mexico chili

- Zedoary

- Mint marigold

- Chives

- Willowherb

- Star anise

- Njangsa

- Sweet woodruff

- Salad burnet

- Mastic

- Cilantro

- Wintergreen

- Fenugreek

- Koseret leaves

- Barberry

- Kokam seed

- Cinnamon, true or Ceylon

- Galingale

- Avocado leaf

- Huacatay, Mexican marigold

- Filé powder, gumbo filé

- Kaffir lime leaves

- Hoja santa

- Ethiopian cardamom

- Paprika

- Hyssop

- Oregano

- Houttuynia cordata

- Nutmeg

- Elderflower

- Kawakawa seeds

- Poppyseed

- Pandan flower

- Musk mallow

- Red rice powder

- Yarrow

- Spearmint

- Mustard plant

- Watercress

- Sorrel

- Sesame Seed

- Pennyroyal

- Alkanet

- Carom seeds

- Sage

- Alexanders

- Basil, sweet

- Tarragon

- Bay leaf

- Mountain Horopito Spikenard

- Savory, summer

- Ajwain

- Turmeric

- Aniseed myrtle

- Catnip

- Wormwood

- Solanum centrale

- Pandan leaf

- Angelica

- Alligator pepper

- Anise

- Clove

- Cudweed

- Marjoram

- Ginger, torch

- Akudjura

- Grains of paradise

- Caper

- Chicory

- Cinnamon, Saigon, or Vietnamese

- Chinese black cardamom

- California Bay laurel

- Fennel

- Caraway

- Cao Guo

- Costmary

- Cardamom

- Clary sage

- Cardamom, black

- Coriander seed

- Grains of Selim

Edible Seeds

Edible seeds are suitable for both animal and human consumption, and different plants produce them. Seeds are the most dominant source of protein and calories. Most plants that produce seeds are angiosperms, while others are gymnosperms. The most important types of seeds are cereals, legumes, and nuts. Legumes and cereals correspond with plants that belong to botanical families.

Grains (Millets and Cereals)

Grains are edible seeds of plants or grass and belong to the Poaceae family. There are two main varieties of grains, including cereals produced by drought-sensitive crops, and millets that are small and drought resistant. There are different ways to eat grains, but most require husking and cooking. They can also be ground into flour and constitute staple food in many societies. Cereals also provide the majority of calories to consumers. The following are the common types of cereals and grains.

- Sorghum

- Asia rice

- Teff

- Finger millet

- Wild rice

- African rice

- Black and white fonio

- Corn, maize, corn kernel

- Little and pearl millet

- Kernza

- Emma, Kamut

- Rye

- Wheat

- Barley

- Groat

- Foxtail millet

- Triticale

Other grasses that provide edible seeds include woollybutt grass, barley Mitchel grass, wattle signalgrass, bunch panic, and kangaroo grass.

Legumes

A legume is the edible seed of a plant belonging to the family Fabaceae. Legumes can be divided into dals that split and grams that do not split. The following are examples of legumes.

- Groundnuts

- Black gram

- Lima bean

- Indian beechnut

- Chickpea, garbanzo bean

- Mung bean

- Bambara groundnut

- Pigeon pea

- Adzuki bean

- Fava bean, broad bean

- Soybean

- Lentil

- Common bean

- Pea

- Cowpea

- Green gram

There are different types of beans, and some can be consumed raw while others need to be cooked before consumption.

Culinary Nuts

Nuts constitute a particular type of fruit according to the botanical definition. For instance, chestnuts, acorns, and hazelnuts are examples of nuts under this category. However, the term also includes other fruits that do not qualify as botanical nuts but offer a similar culinary role and appearance. The following are examples of culinary nuts.

Types of Chestnuts

- Acorn

- Almond

- Beech

- Brazil nut

- Candlenut

- Cashew

- Chinese chestnuts

- Chilean hazel

- Squash seeds

- Guinea peanuts

- Hazelnuts

- Kola nut

- Macadamia

- Malaba almond

- Hickory

- Mamoncillo

- Mongongo

- Ogbono

- Paradise nut

- Pili

- Pistachio

- Shear nut

- Walnuts

- Black walnut

- Melon seeds

- Sweet chestnuts

- Japanese chestnuts

Other Edible Seeds

The following are other types of edible seeds that do not belong to the categories mentioned above.

- Chempedak

- Coffee bean

- Cocoa bean

- Durian

- Fox nut

- Hemp seed

- Jackfruit

- Lotus seed

- Mustard seed

- Sunflower seed

- Poppyseed

- Pumpkin seed

- Watermelon seed

- Pomegranate seed

Nut-like Gymnosperm Seeds

The following are seeds that are similar to nuts.

- Juniper

- Gnetum

- Ginkgo

- Monkey puzzle

- Cycads

- Pine nuts (Korean pine, Pinhao, Mexican pinyon. Chilgoza pine, Pinon pine)

Edible Flowers

Different types of flowers can be consumed raw or cooked. Other flowers can be dried and added to various dishes for flavoring or coloring. However, you need to know the appropriate recipe if you want to enjoy your food. The following are good examples of consumable flowers.

- Chervil

- Cornflower

- Rose

- Rosemary

- Tulip

- Daisy

- Sacred flower

- Chamomile

- Geranium

- French marigold

- Asparagus

- Chrysanthemum

- Chinese hibiscus

- Mint

- Pansy

- Marigold

- Chicory

- Sunflower

- Passionflower

- Common dandelion

- Dill

- Squash

- Woodruff

- Bergamot

- Red clover

- Snapdragon

- Purple bauhinia, butterfly tree

- Fennel

- Common bean

- Thyme

- Starflower

- orchid tree

- Daylily

- Common violet

- Linden

- Marshmallow plant

- Cabbage

- Lavender

- Common sage

- Pineapple sage

- Chives

- Carnation

- Lovage

- Lilac

- Heart's ease

- Okra

- Arugula

- Basil

- Japanese honeysuckle

- Indian cress

Leafy Vegetables

Leafy vegetables are primarily grown for consumption, but some are cultivated for medicinal purposes. For example, vegetables like lime have medicinal properties, and others are infused in tea. There are several types of leaf vegetables, and the following are some of them.

- Indian mustard

- Climbing wattle

- African cabbage

- Mountain sorrel

- Burnet Saxifrage

- Sensitive fern

- Broad-leaved Plantain

- Cinnamon fern

- Japanese Red Pine

- Queensland grass-cloth plant

- Cauliflower

- Pheka

- Myrobalan

- Tree lettuce

- Garden pea

- Radish

- Seven Sisters Rose

- Primrose

- French Scorzonera

- Buckshorn plantain

- Indian spinach

- American Wormseed

- Rough fogfruit

- Terebinth

- Water Lettuce

- Raffia palm

- Cowslip

- Lesser celandine

- Meadow beauty

- American Bistort

- Common Marshmallow

- Lima Bean

- Mexican pepper leaf

- Common evening primrose

- John's Cabbage

- West African pepper

- Cha-phlu

- Chinese Pistache

- Kerguelen cabbage

- Long-leaved plantain

- Abyssinian Cabbage

- Aniseed

- Knotweed

- Birch-Leaved Pear

- Chinese radish

- Sorrel

- Palm-grass

- Sow Thistle

- Alsike Clover

- Wild radish

- Kale

- Lemon basil

- Prairie turnip

- Elephant Bush

- Ethiopian moringa

- Lungwort

- Benniseed

- Chayote

- Rose crown

- Salad Burnet

- Black Mustard

- Star Gooseberry

- Weeping Willow

- Alpine bistort

- Eastern Swamp Saxifrage

- Blackcurrant

- Creeping Rockfoil

- Opposite leaved saltwort

- Spreading stonecrop

- Bistort

- Wild Cabbage

- Broad-leaved endive

- Interrupted fern

- Blue Palo Verde

- Oca

- Arctic butterbur

- Water pepper

- Money tree

- Sea daisy

- Common wood sorrel

- Cabbage

- Sugarloaf

- Perilla

- Petai

- Runner Bean

- Parsnip

- Round-headed rampion

- Golden lace

- Common Reed

- Creeping wood sorrel

- Turnip

- Himalayan mayapple

- Barbados Gooseberry

- Burra Gookeroo

- American Pokeweed

- Runner Bean

- Clearweed

- Bella Sombra

- Deer calalu

- Indian Pokeberry

- Brussels Sprouts

- Curly endive

- Oak-Leaved Goosefoot

- Parrot feather

- Celtuce

- Hooker's Evening-primrose

- Empress tree

- Phak chet

- Tatsoi

- Iron Cross

- Mizuna

- Radicchio

- Dittander

- Maca

- Watercress

- Water Celery

- Cicely

- Redwood sorrel

- Parsley

- Common yellow wood sorrel

- Common amaranth

- Rampion

- Water Spinach

- Sweet Potato

- Samphire

- Dragon's head

- Henbit deadnettle

- Hawkbit

- Bottle Gourd

- Musk Mallow

- Purple amaranth

- Catsear

- Quinoa

- Prickly Lettuce

- Rice paddy herb, Ngò om

- Kogomi

- Drumstick tree

- Ice plant

- South-west African moringa

- Fragrant Water Lily

- Paracress

- Nipplewort

- Cheeseweed

- Habek mint

- Southern Huauzontle

- Mauka

- Sweet Basil

- Water Snowflake

- Thai basil

- Yellow floating heart

- Sea Beet

- Kuḷḷafila

- Mallow

- Japanese mint

- Sea bluebell

- Cassava

- Seep monkeyflower

- Red deadnettle

- Noni tree

- Wall lettuce

- Celery

- Napa Cabbage

- Garland chrysanthemum

- Lacinato kale

- White deadnettle

- Golden samphire

- Garden cress

- Virginia pepperweed

- Gooseneck Loosestrife

- Field pepperweed

- Slender amaranth

- Rapini

- Cabbage thistle

- Lablab

- Spotted Cat's-ear

- Indian Lettuce

- Bush Banana

- Phak kratin

- Genjer

- Lovage

- Garden orache

- Lamb's Quarters

- Good King Henry

- Asian pennywort

- Siberian spring beauty

- Gotukola

- Red Goosefoot

- Endive

- Miner's lettuce

- Mitsuba

- Prickly amaranth

- Broccoli

- Belgian endive

- Wild Coxcomb

- Sea kale

- Amaranth

- Huauzontle

- Chipilín

- Chaya or tree spinach

- Jew's mallow

- Chik-nam, Kra don

- Harebell

- Tree Spinach

- Chicory

- Redflower ragleaf

- Puntarelle

- Caigua

- Taro

- Phak tiu som or Phak tiu daeng

- Ivy Gourd

- Common Borage

- Chinese Savoy

- Bok Choi

- Caper

- Gallant Soldier

- Cilantro

- Coriander

- Lotus sweet juice

- Melindjo

- Okinawan Spinach

- Chard

- Lettuce

- Covo

- Viagra palm

- Ground Ivy

- Arugula

- Rocket

- Bhandhanya

- Culantro

- Elecampane

- Bank cress

- Kai-lan

- Rape Kale

- Beet, Beetroot

- Sea purslane

- Lesser jack

- Roselle

- Shawnee Salad

- Fennel

- Shortpod mustard

- Rutabaga

- Spinach

- Komatsuna

- Cardoon

- Perennial Wall-rocket

- Thong lang

- Sea sandwort

- Scarlina

- Fishwort

- Vegetable fern

Edible Mushrooms

Mushrooms are a fleshy species of macro-fungi that produce large edible structures. They are commonly found above the ground though some grow below the ground, and they are picked by hand. Edible mushrooms have a desirable aroma and taste and also have a nutritional value, and they can be cultivated or harvested wild.

However, other types of mushrooms can be highly poisonous, so you need to be well informed in identifying them. Other types of mushrooms can cause allergic reactions. Great care should be taken when preparing the fungus for consumption. The following are common types of edible mushrooms.

- Chanterelle (Girolle) Mushrooms

- Button (White) Mushrooms

- Oyster Mushrooms

- Shimeji Mushroom

- Enoki (Snow Puff) Mushrooms

- Cremini (Italian Brown) Mushrooms

- Parasol Mushroom

- Shiitake (Forest or Oak) Mushrooms

- Portobello (Portabella) Mushrooms

- Porcini (Cepe or Bolete) Mushrooms

- Crab Brittlegill Mushroom

- Straw Mushroom

- Black Trumpet Mushroom

- Chicken of the Woods Mushroom

- Button Mushroom

- Morel Mushroom

- Charcoal Burner Mushroom

- Common Ink Cap Mushroom

- Cremini Mushroom

- Bay Bolete Mushroom

- Chanterelle Mushroom

- Cauliflower Mushroom

- Shiitake Mushroom

- Enoki Mushroom

- False Morel Mushroom

- Wood Blewit Mushroom

- Field Mushroom

- King Oyster Mushroom

- Dryad's Saddle

- Yellow Knight Mushroom

- Morel Mushrooms

- Hedgehog Mushroom

- Giant Puffball Mushroom

- Reishi Mushroom

- Honey Fungus Mushroom

- Gypsy Mushroom

- King Bolete Mushroom

- Green Cracking Russula

- Matsutake Mushroom

- Wood Ear Mushroom

- Portobello Mushroom

- Slippery Jack Mushroom

- Caesar's Mushroom

- Maitake Mushroom

- Red Pine Mushroom

- Lion's Mane Mushroom

Apart from the potential toxins and allergic reactions that some types of mushrooms can cause, the edible ones are good for you. They have nutrients and phytochemicals that are not readily available in fruits, vegetables, and meat. Additionally, mushrooms are fat-free, contain several antioxidants, and are high in fiber, copper, B vitamins, and potassium.

What Are the Differences between Plants, Flowers, and Weeds?

Plants are grown intentionally in the fields and gardens. They are harvested for consumption when they are ripe. All other unwanted plants that grow in the garden are called weeds. Weeds grow rapidly and produce large quantities of seeds often blown by the wind or transported by animals. Weeds are resistant to natural forces and can grow in diverse habitats. Herbicides control weeds, but these can affect other plants and the environment. Other controls are to manually remove weeds or mulch your garden. Most plants produce flowers that will develop into seeds or edible products. Many people grow flowers to improve the appearance of their homes.

You can grow wild edible plants in your garden, but there are different things you should know. Wild plants can adapt to specific conditions, so it's necessary to first understand your climate and environment. It is a good idea to take your soil for testing to know if it is suitable for the specific types of plants you want to grow. You should also know the time it takes to grow plants until they are ready for harvesting. Storage is another crucial aspect you must know about if you decide to venture into the farming of edible plants.

People obtain their food from different sources. Since time memorial, people have been foraging for edible plants for their survival, and these come in various forms. In this chapter, we have discussed different types of edible plants. These plants offer a variety of nutrients, and they can be consumed raw or cooked. Before eating these plants and flowers, make sure they are not poisonous. Another essential element is knowing how to grow, harvest, store, and prepare various forms of plants if you want to enjoy their nutritional value.

Chapter 2: Benefits of Eating Edible Wild Plants

In recent years, more and more people have been adopting healthier choices in their diet. Eating and growing organic foods are on the rise because of their sustainability and health benefits. This practice also supports local growers and farmers and contributes to the community as a whole. But not everyone has access to organic and local produce because of their location or the high cost of these plants. This chapter will discuss the various benefits of eating edible wild plants and mention edible plant parts.

Health Benefits

Research has shown that eating different varieties of plants is extremely beneficial to the gut microbiota. If you consume over 30 varieties every week, you'll absorb plenty of antioxidants that promote better health as they neutralize free radicals or waste products produced in the body. If free radicals are not removed from the body, they produce oxidative stress, increasing the risk of heart disease, respiratory diseases, immune deficiency, stroke, cancer, and arthritis, to name a few.

Antioxidants like vitamins A, C, and E, manganese, beta-carotene, lutein, and selenium remove free radicals from the body. These are found in numerous edible wild plants like elderberries, huckleberry, gooseberries, mulberries, leeks, onions, garlic, carrots, pumpkin, spinach, and mangoes. Eating different plant varieties can decrease the incidence of hypertension, diabetes, and heart diseases. Ensure your diet contains various types and colors to obtain a mixture of nutrients essential for your body. Your meals will look brighter and more appetizing, and you'll be getting plenty of health benefits as well.

Many wild plants play a major role in reducing chronic inflammation and arthritic pain. Your body produces inflammation as a normal immune response for self-healing. However, too much inflammation can cause significant damage. Wild plants like the stinging nettle, elderberry, and curly dock can block the production of inflammatory hormones in the body and aid in pain relief for chronic inflammatory conditions. Its anti-inflammatory and antihistaminic properties as provided in the high flavonoid and antioxidant content.

We all suffer from digestive problems from time to time. Whether it's from eating sugary and fatty foods or eating too many complex fibers, sometimes our digestive tract can't break down food properly. When this happens, your body responds by making you feel bloated or constipated. These symptoms of indigestion indicate an f inflammation in your digestive tract. Your body gets inflamed because your immune system is trying to protect your digestive system. Apart from eating unhealthy foods, indigestion can also be caused by chronic stress and anxiety. While some medicines can relieve flatulence, constipation, heartburn, or other forms of indigestion, they only treat the symptoms and not the problem itself. Most heartburn medicines treat inflammation but hinder digestion as well, which adds to your digestive discomfort.

A great alternative is eating some edible wild plants that work to give you a healthy digestive tract and aid in digestion. Wild fennel is one of these plants and can be found in many areas of the United States. It has carminative properties that aid in digestion and relieve flatulence and constipation. Fennel seeds can be eaten raw or cooked with your meals. You can also make fennel tea, which you can enjoy after your meals to improve digestion.

Rosemary can be found abundantly in the wild and is easily identified because of its distinctive smell and shape. Its antioxidant properties reduce inflammation and promote a healthy gut.

Chamomile is another great wild plant to aid digestion. It also helps to reduce stress as its carminative properties can relax your muscles. It's recommended to drink chamomile tea after meals to improve digestion and before going to bed to improve sleep quality.

It is also known some wild plants decrease hypertension. This common condition is a major concern, as it increases the risk of strokes and heart disease. Some wild plants have certain characteristics that relieve hypertension. For example, stinging nettle can activate nitric oxide production in the body. Nitric oxide is a vasodilator that widens blood vessels, which relieves hypertension. It also contains other compounds that mimic the action of calcium channel blockers. This action indirectly lowers high blood pressure as it relaxes the heart and decreases the force of its contractions.

Another great wild plant is the crowd-favorite asparagus, used in many recipes. It is rich in potassium, which widens the blood vessels and removes excess salt from the body. Raspberries are another wild plant rich in potassium. Raspberry also contains omega-3 fatty acids that reduce the incidence of strokes and heart disease. This delicious and succulent fruit has numerous additional benefits - from managing diabetes, high cholesterol, and high blood pressure. Its high fiber and low sugar content help to increase the feeling of satiety, which is why it is recommended for weight loss.

Wild garlic mustard makes a flavorful addition to your recipes and has numerous health benefits. Many people are concerned about its rapid growth because it's considered invasive. A great way to control its spread is by simply picking it and adding it to your recipes. Garlic mustard has a distinctive and strong taste of garlic that enriches your sauces, soups, vegetables, and proteins. It is a versatile plant that has many uses.

Regarding its medicinal value, garlic mustard has numerous health benefits. The whole plant can be used to improve blood circulation in the body. When blood flows smoothly throughout the body, coordination between the different organs and tissues is at peak condition. This coordination promotes cell regeneration and overall health. You can use the leaves of the garlic mustard plant in your green smoothies to give it an extra spicy kick. The leaves can be dried and seasoned, and added to your dishes for flavor. They are rich in vitamins A and C and other minerals. The roots make a great addition to soups and can also be salted or pickled as it has a potent flavor characterized with spicy and peppery notes similar to wasabi or horseradish. A great advantage about garlic mustard is you can use its flowers, roots, greens, and seeds in your salads, smoothies, soups, and main dishes. Its versatility and abundance in the wild make it one of the most common edible wild plants.

Dandelions are another great example of a wild plant with health benefits. Like garlic mustard, the whole plant can be consumed from root to flower. It is a highly nutritious plant packed with minerals, vitamins, and fibers. The younger leaves can be eaten raw, but the mature leaves become bitter, so it's best to boil them first. You can add them to your salads and other dishes as a garnish for their bright color and earthy, nutty flavor. The flowers can also be used similarly in salads for added color and flavor. The leaves are rich in vitamins A, C, and K, minerals like potassium, magnesium, iron, and calcium. The roots contain high levels of inulin, a carbohydrate that promotes healthy gut microbiota.

Like most wild plants, dandelions are rich in antioxidants, which reduce chronic inflammation in the body. They also contain bioactive compounds that lower blood sugar levels. They work on the absorption of glucose levels in the muscles and stimulate the release of insulin to regulate blood sugar levels. Other compounds in the plant can lower cholesterol in the blood, which decreases the risk of heart disease.

Dandelion tea is recommended for people with hypertension due to its diuretic effect. This action helps remove toxins and excess fluids from the body, which helps relieve hypertension. Its high potassium content indirectly lowers blood pressure by getting rid of excess salt through urine. Since dandelions can decrease fats in the body, they can prevent liver damage and help with weight management. This wild plant has other numerous benefits, including preventing indigestion, boosting immunity, and promoting healthy skin by decreasing the incidence of acne, fine wrinkles, and sun damage.

Discovering New Ingredients

When eating edible wild plants, you'll discover a whole new world of ingredients to add to your food every day. You'll learn to become creative with your recipes and explore new tastes, encouraging you to make meals diverse and enjoy different foods in your diet. Edible wild plants cannot be found in your typical farmer's market or grocery store. This makes them a great addition to your dishes, reviving old and dull recipes. You can use them as a garnish for your salads and main dishes or as a primary ingredient. This will encourage you to cultivate your foraging habit as you discover new foods daily.

Managing Invasive Plants

Invasive plants are nonnative species that can grow rapidly under the right environmental conditions. Their growth is problematic because they crowd out native plants and disrupt their ecosystems. Not all invasive plants are easily spotted, as sometimes you can hardly differentiate between them and native plants. With time and practice, you'll learn which plants in your area are invasive and which of those are edible.

Invasive plants are spread by humans or animals transporting seeds to different areas. If you plant a native plant in your garden, dogs, squirrels, or other animals may carry its seeds or dry fruits in their fur and move them to another area. They grow and spread rapidly in that area, taking over the land where other native plant species grow. This makes them invasive plants, which may appear beautiful but are harmful to native plant communities.

Some nonnative plant species are not invasive. A plant must exhibit rapid growth in a foreign environment to be classified as invasive. It has to outgrow native plants easily and thrive in its new environment. Rose bushes and Japanese oak are examples of nonnative noninvasive plants that could grow in your garden. They don't spread aggressively enough to hinder the growth of other native plants.

Apart from rapid and aggressive growth, a lack of natural predators also contributes to the spread of invasive plants. Most of these plants have an unpalatable taste that doesn't appeal to wild animals. They are resilient and can withstand severe damage from fires, cutting, and uprooting. Many of them can even grow from broken roots that were improperly cut in an attempt to control them. Some types even survive certain types of poison, which makes them extremely dangerous to wild animals and plants.

A great way to eliminate invasive plants is to eat the edible varieties. As we've said, a surprising number are edible and can add a delicious flavor to your meals. For example, knotweed shoots can be peeled and added raw or pickled to salads or grilled and sauteed and added to soups, pies, chutneys, and even main dishes. Other invasive plants include wild watercress, autumn berries, aggressive onion, and mugwort. These varieties have their popularity has been on the rise recently thanks to conservation foraging, where many gatherers concentrate on more sustainable harvesting strategies. Nowadays, many chefs incorporate invasive plants that were once considered weeds and thrown away in their recipes.

Discovering Local and Sacred Plants

Eating edible wild plants is a great way to learn about local plants in your area. You'll learn how to identify different species of plants and find ways to use them in your cooking. Sacred plants can be found in the wild and contain medicinal characteristics. Ancient cultures have used them for hundreds of years to relieve different ailments. You need to familiarize yourself with the different sacred plants found in the world before foraging them.

Many cultures consider a plant sacred if people can incorporate it into food. Common examples in North and Central America include corn and wild rice. The Great Lakes region in North America is home to the Ojibwe people, who believe wild rice or "manoomin" to be a sacred plant. The Great Lakes hold a vast land of wild rice, widely used in Native American cuisine. Corn is also considered a sacred plant in Native American culture as it has been a primary ingredient in their cuisine for thousands of years. You can still find corn stalks in the wild growing in large groups.

Most medicines were originally derived from plants, so many cultures consider certain varieties sacred. These plants are found in the wild and can be easily identified and used to relieve certain symptoms. However, it's important to consult your doctor before you attempt to use these varieties. You also need to ensure uprooting or cutting certain plants is allowed because it may be offensive to some cultures. St. John's Wort is one of the most common sacred plants found in the wild. Its use for medicinal purposes was famous among Early European pagans and Christians. This sacred plant was used as an antidepressant and calmative agent. It was also believed to ward off evil forces.

Sweetgrass is another sacred plant with a sweet aroma. It has anticoagulant properties but can be harmful to the liver if abused. Many people place it in their homes for its warm vanilla-like scent and use it to add a distinctive flavor to foods and beverages. It can also be used indoors as a mosquito repellent. Ginger and papaya are great examples of wild scared plants with medicinal properties as they both can relieve nausea. Other plants like garlic and pineapple reduce inflammation and pain from bee stings and mosquito bites.

You can find epazote growing in the wild in southern regions of the United States, Mexico, and Central America. It has a pungent smell that some associate with gasoline, while others describe it as sweet and citrusy. Epazote is added to beans for flavor and as an anti-flatulent agent. It is also known to fight off parasites in the digestive tract and repel mosquitoes and other insects. Mullein is another sacred medicinal plant found in most regions of the United States. This plant can also be found in countries with temperate climates. It's used to treat earaches and mild respiratory distress.

Getting in Touch with Nature

Nowadays, many people suffer from nature-deficit syndrome. They become more disconnected from nature, spending most of their time working from home. Some people don't find hiking in nature fun, but it becomes an entertaining activity if you combine walking or hiking with foraging for wild plants. You can make a whole day out of it with your friends and family.

Make the day interesting by arranging a competition to see which one gathers the most edible varieties and finds the unique plants.

Doing physical activity outdoors is a great way to exercise. When you combine physical exercise with the mental activity needed for foraging, you will begin to feel more grounded and closer to your roots. Modern-day technology has been distancing us from nature, which is the source of our existence. Nature brings us food for sustenance, but it also connects us with who we are. When you take a hike in the wild, you discover new plant species every day, and you become acquainted with wildflowers, fruits, and vegetables, many of which are edible and contain higher nutrients than store-bought produce.

When you pick your own food, you start to feel more independent and freer. You get to appreciate your food sources, which make you more conscious about the environment and sustainable practices. Foraging is beneficial to individuals, but it can help a whole community make smarter choices about the environment on a larger scale. In this day and age, environmental issues have become prominent more than ever. It's important to get in touch with nature so that you know what's at stake. You may have heard about why it's important to make sustainable choices, but unless you regularly get in touch with nature, you won't take the right step toward sustainability.

Getting your hands dirty while foraging is a great way to appreciate the farmers and gatherers who work hard from early morning until noon, sometimes under the scorching sun, to harvest their crops and get them to the grocery stores and your table. Imagine deleting all those steps by merely taking a nature walk and picking some delicious food ingredients to use in your cooking.

When you connect with the sun, wind, rain, and the soil in the earth, you don't just connect with nature. You feel the symbiotic relationship between different plants and how they are affected by animals and insects. You will feel more bonded with nature, and you'll get excited at the thought of picking your own foods.

Saving Money

Picking and eating edible plants has a great economic advantage. It's no secret that organic produce is usually quite expensive. Most of your meals depended on fruits and vegetables on a plant-based diet. Your grocery bill would be steep, and sometimes you may get bored from eating the same plants repeatedly. Foraging allows you to explore various plant sources without breaking the bank. While you may not live next to an area where you can forage, you can still make the best of your trip by gathering fruits that you can freeze for months, s like most types of wild berries.

Eating Healthier and More Sustainable Foods

Ecology is another plus for changing to a plant-based diet and using edible wild plants. First of all, you are guaranteed to collect 100% organic plants free from pesticides and fertilizers. People have been developing ways to domesticate plants and shape modern-day agricultural strategies for thousands of years. By the dawn of the Industrial Age, many harmful practices were introduced, including using chemical pesticides and fertilizers. The widespread use of these chemicals caused the detrimental impact we suffer from to this day.

Fertilizers are used to provide essential nutrients for growing and developing plants. When plants are uprooted, cut, or harvested repeatedly, the nutrients in the soil become depleted. Fertilizers are then added to replenish lost nutrients. It's better to use organic fertilizers, which mainly consist of animal manure and other composted materials that facilitate plants' growth. The nutrients in chemical fertilizers are limited to three: minerals, potassium, nitrogen, and phosphorus. While these fertilizers promote growth, they are not as diverse as organic fertilizers containing an abundance of different nutrients like calcium, magnesium, and iron, among many others.

Chemical fertilizers can also contaminate water streams and promote the growth of algae that take over the water surface and prevent oxygen from passing through to the fish species living underneath. Overfertilization using synthetic fertilizers leads to a dangerous accumulation of nutrients, which alters the pH of the soil and damages the plants.

When it comes to using chemical pesticides, the disadvantages outweigh the advantages. For one, pesticides don't just kill harmful organisms that damage crops. They kill even the useful organisms that promote the mineralization of nutrients in the soil, release plant hormones, and help to fight pests. Pesticides are also harmful to people who use them on their crops, consume foods exposed to them, or live near agricultural areas. Another major disadvantage of pesticides is most pests have become immune to them. Studies have found that more crops are damaged today due to pests compared to the mid-1900s.

These problems created by chemicals sprayed on crops are not found with wild plants. They don't need to be watered, cultivated, or fertilized. The beauty of wild plants is that nature takes care of them. They are the ultimate natural product offering the healthiest, most sustainable produce. They can be found growing abundantly in farms, gardens, and even sidewalks. Since these plants are unaltered, you will notice that they taste much better than any type of domesticated plant.

Which Plant Parts Are Edible?

Identifying which plant parts are edible requires a knowledge of the plant's anatomy. Plants consist of roots, stems, leaves, and branches which carry the fruits and flowers. These parts are an invaluable reservoir for starch and essential nutrients needed for growth and development. The plant's reproductive organs are the fruits and flowers, which carry the plant's seeds or embryo. The seeds are extracted from these fruits and flowers by insects, animals, or humans and planted in the soil to produce more plants. Other plant parts protect these organs to preserve the most valued part, which is the seed.

All these plant parts contain a high amount of fiber. There are two kinds of fiber: water-soluble or insoluble. Fiber is one of the most useful aids in digestion and toxin and waste elimination from the body. Fruits and vegetables are classified into roots, stems, leaves, fruits, flowers, and seeds. Fruits are the plants' ovaries in their mature state. Vegetables are divided into roots, leaves, stems, shoots, tubers, and other parts. Some vegetables are considered root vegetables like beetroots, but their leaves can also be used in various food recipes.

Let's look at the different types of fruits, vegetables, and seeds we eat and the categories they fall under. Wheat, corn, wheat, wild rice, maize, mustard, soybean, hemp seeds, flax seeds, and peas, for instance, are considered seeds. Root vegetables grow underground to absorb nutrients from the soil. Examples include potatoes, carrots, turnips, radishes, and beetroots.

Some plants' edible parts are the stems or stalks, which is the main body part of the plant. These include asparagus, rhubarb, celery, broccoli, and spinach. Leafy vegetables include parsley, dill, cilantro, spinach, cabbage, and Swiss chard. Fruits contain seeds and are usually sweet and starchy, or succulent and fleshy, like apples, bananas, orange, tangerine, tomato, and pumpkin. Flowers are typically colorful and also bear the seeds of the plant. Examples include zucchini flowers, cauliflower, broccoli, and spices like cinnamon and cloves.

Now, let's take a look at some common wild plants for foraging and the parts you can use in your recipes. You can find many bamboo species in the wild with flavors ranging from sweet to savory. The shoots are the only edible part of the plants, and they need to be boiled before consumption. You have to identify the right type of bamboo for eating as some types have a high cyanogenic glycoside content, which is toxic if consumed at high levels. Blueberries are one of the most common berries to find in the wild. The fruits are the edible part of the plant, but make sure to distinguish them from other similar-looking poisonous berries.

The prickly pear cactus is another sweet and succulent fruit found in the wild. It is vibrant color varying from red and purple to yellow. The green fruits are unripe, so make sure you only pick the colorful ones, which will be sweeter and softer. Be careful when you peel the skin because spikes surround it. Kelp is a great source of fiber and can be eaten whole, with some parts being more palatable than others. Avoid eating kelp growing in industrial areas or washed up on shores because they may be rotten or toxic.

While picking wild mushrooms requires some expertise to avoid poisonous varieties, you'd be lucky to find lobster mushrooms as you hike through temperate forests across northern regions of the US. These mushrooms can be eaten whole. They have a sweet, nutty flavor that many people associate with poached lobster, which makes a delicious treat if you're hiking in the wild.

In this chapter, we discussed the benefits of eating edible plants, from absorbing their various nutrients to making eco-friendly choices, and how important it is to be able to identify each plant correctly. We'll discuss which types of wild plants are poisonous to watch out for in the following chapters. Remember, some edible wild plants might cause allergic reactions, so make sure to test them carefully before consumption.

Chapter 3: Understanding Foraging

Foraging is the act of searching for food in the wild. It's a basic survival mechanism of wildlife - one you'll have to learn if you're about to go searching for wild edibles. That said, foraging is as complicated as it sounds. There are a lot of things you should consider and many rules to follow. If this is your first adventure in the wild, here's everything you need to know about foraging.

How to Identify an Edible Wild Plant

To get started, you must first learn the basic surviving mechanisms in the wild. The best option is to have enough knowledge and experience to identify the wild plants you come across, but what if you can't do that for one reason or another? In that case, you'll need to rely on the universal edibility test.

The US Army's survival experts have devised this test. Although it takes a long time to yield results (about 24 hours), it's your best bet for staying strong and healthy. Here are the steps you should follow:

1.   Begin by fasting for eight hours, during which you can only drink fresh water.

2.   Divide the plant according to its parts: flowers, buds, leaves, stems, and roots. Only test one part at a time.

3.   Smell each part, and discard the plant if it smells rotten, musty, or unpleasant odor. Throw it away instantly if you smell anything like almonds or pears, which can indicate cyanide.

4.   Place a part of the plant on the inner side of your elbow to test for contact poisoning. Keep it there for eight hours and throw it away if you feel your skin burning, itching, going numb, or breaking out in a rash. Wash your elbow right away in that case.

5.   If there is no contact poisoning, prepare another small part of the plant for eating. To be safe, it's always better to boil it first.

6.   Touch the plant to your lips first before taking a bite, and if your lips start itching or burning, throw it away.

7.   If you wait for 15 minutes without getting any reaction, take a small bite, chew, and hold it in your mouth for another 15 minutes. Spit it out if you feel a soapy or bitter taste, and wash out your mouth.

8.   If all goes well, you can assume the plant is safe to eat but swallow the first bite and wait for another eight hours.

9.   If you don't suffer from any side effects, you can confirm the plant is edible. You can then repeat the test for other parts.

10.   Don't use this test to identify mushrooms, as they don't work the same way other plants do.

Since this test takes a long time, it's best to know in advance the deadliest and most poisonous species in the area to avoid wasting time. Learning the defining features of edible plants is also a great way to minimize confusion.

Foraging 101: Rules for the Beginner

Learning how to identify edible plants is one of the most basic foraging rules, but it doesn't end there. There are a lot of rules when it comes to foraging, and just because a wild plant is available doesn't mean you can, or should, eat it. You'll build up experience the more you go foraging, but for beginners venturing out in the wild for the first time, it's imperative to have some guidelines to show you the ropes. Here's what you need to know.

1. Never Eat What You Don't Know

The first rule is simple: never eat what you don't know. Unless you can be 100% positive of the plant's identity, you should never risk eating it - be it raw or processed. If you have even a shred of doubt, don't eat it. A lot of wild food is downright poisonous, and there are a lot of poisonous lookalikes you can confuse with edible plants.

2. Fortify Your Knowledge

As exciting as it is to venture into the wild on your own, it's also dangerous. Although this sense of danger is what's alluring about foraging, you should be prudent and responsible about approaching a foreign and wild environment. The best thing you can do is to arm yourself with knowledge, and what better way to do that than to find a mentor? An expert will easily guide you through your area of choice and boost your confidence.

Whether you find a mentor or not, it's equally important to increase your knowledge by reading and studying books. Many books about wild edibles can help you identify species and guide you through the best way to eat them. Luckily for you, this is one of those books!

3.   Learn the Latin Names

Learning to identify plants using common names will only take you so far. If you want to be certain about your identification, it's better to learn Latin names. You can never go wrong with Latin names - since it's a dead language, you won't have to worry about the plant name changing or evolving in different areas. You may drink tea brewed from Tsuga canadensis or Eastern Hemlock tree, but drinking Conium maculatum tea, or Poison Hemlock, is an unwise move. Unfortunately, both can be offered as "hemlock tea," but you can save yourself by learning how to differentiate between both species using their Latin names.

4.   Recognize the Edible Parts of Every Species

Just because you stumbled across an edible plant doesn't mean you can consume all of it. Most edible plants are not completely edible; only certain parts are, while the rest are toxic. For instance, you can safely eat elderberries (the fruit), whether raw or cooked, but the same plant's stems, roots, and barks are poisonous. Moreover, it's equally important to note the time of the year in which the edible parts are, well, edible. Stinging nettle is generally safe to eat, but it's not when it goes to seed.

5.   Learn about the Poisonous Local Species

Learning how to identify poisonous species is just as important as identifying edible ones. Before you set out, be sure to make a list of the poisonous species in your area.

6.   Study the Land and Habitat

If you see a yellow dock, there are high chances you'll soon stumble upon pokeweed. That's the reason you need to become familiar with other plants that are known to grow in the same place as the wild edibles you're looking for. When you learn more about the habitat, you'll know that you'll never find ramps in swamps, just like cattails won't grow on a high slope. Learning about the land you're visiting and studying its wildlife habitat will gain you a whole new experience. You'll learn to watch the behavior of the animals and insects and understand not just their foraging behavior but also their lifestyles. This will help you find the food crops and make you feel like you're a part of a bigger ecosystem.

7.   Recognize the Trees

Just like you can learn to pinpoint wild edibles from their companion plants, you can find them by scrutinizing the trees in the area. As it happens, most wild edibles only grow in areas that receive full sunlight. The surrounding trees will also help to guide you to your edibles. If your edibles prefer acidic tracts of land, as wild berries do, look for conifer trees like spruce or pine. You can look for cypress and juniper trees to find large-scale blueberry crops, which are otherwise only found in small amounts.

8.   Forage within Your Borders

Wild edibles are available for the taking by anyone, but that's not the case on privately-owned or protected properties. Before you start wondering about an isolated place, make sure it's available for the public. Ask around and get permission before wandering the premises if you're unsure.

9.   Keep an Eye Out for Hazards

Unfortunately, it's a dangerous world out there - and we're not just talking about wildlife or poisonous plant species. Many wild edibles are no longer edible due to the environmental pollution they suffer through. Before you forage through a land, be sure the plants haven't been sprayed with pesticides or herbicides. If you notice the tree leaves graying or wilting, it's better to steer away from that area. Likewise, never eat any plants growing from a pile of refuse.

Moreover, be sure to equip yourself with proper protective gear when you're out in the wild. For starters, a sturdy pair of hiking shoes will go a very long way - and better get them waterproof if you'll be walking through swamps. Wear a good hat to protect your face and neck from the direct sunlight, get gloves for protecting your hands, and always carry a first-aid kit with you. Don't forget your water bottle to stay hydrated.

10.   Remember, You're Not Alone

It's easy to forget when you're in the middle of nowhere, but you're not alone. You have competition that's also aiming for the wild edibles, so stay alert. Bears will probably be your biggest competitors, but you should also watch out for squirrels and other tiny creatures. If you're not careful, they'll beat you to the nuts.

11.   Use Your Senses

Don't handicap yourself by relying on visual ID alone; many plants have various lookalikes, after all. Instead, learn to differentiate between plants by texture, smell, and other habitat clues. That said, never rely on your sense of taste when identifying your edibles; even a small dose of a poisonous plant can be deadly.

12.   Follow the Lifecycle of Wild Edibles through the Seasons

Learning the lifecycle of your edibles during each season can literally be a life-saver, not to mention, save you a lot of trouble. For instance, beginners can easily mistake poisonous white snakeroot for wood nettle, but anyone can easily tell the difference if the white snakeroots bloom in July. Learning to spot the differences is a great start, but you should also learn to recognize each plant throughout its various stages to avoid making deadly mistakes.

Moreover, learning the lifecycle of plants during the seasons will help you locate the perennial plants you will want to harvest early on in the season. For instance, pokeweed often becomes identifiable during the warmer months, but it's technically inedible at that point. If you make a note of its location during those months, you can easily harvest your fill during early spring when it's less identifiable.

13.   Keep a Foraging Journal

You'll go through a lot of experiences on your foraging journey. You'll make a lot of mistakes, but you'll also unravel wonderful discoveries. As you grow and widen your experience, keep track of everything you've gone through. By keeping a foraging journal to document your experience and growth, you'll have a record of all the wild edibles in your area. This will give you a foraging calendar for your area, so you can plan your foraging adventures.

Essential Gathering Tools

Even veteran foragers need a set of tools to make their job easier. You can't expect to pick up everything by hand or carry your harvest in your pockets. Before you go foraging, here's a complete list of the tools you might possibly need on your journey.

1.   Pruners

Pruners will be one of the tools you'll use the most throughout foraging. You'll need it both when you're gathering and processing herbs, as they snip right through almost everything. If you can only get one tool, choose the highest-quality brand pruners you can afford, so they last for a while. Better yet, get a brand that allows you to replace the blade and spring instead of having to buy new ones every once in a while.

2.   Kitchen Scissors

Pruners, although dependable, do a terrible job when handling delicate greens. They're only suitable for tough stems, and their blade isn't long enough to reach longer stems. If you want to forage for tender-stemmed greens while keeping them intact, you'd better use kitchen scissors. You'll be able to use kitchen scissors to harvest many young greens, like violet, chickweed, and cleavers.

3.   Sharp Compact Knife

You'll also do well with having a compact knife with a sheath on hand, or you can just go for a large folding knife of good quality. You'll use either kind of knife to peel the bark of medicinal trees, so make sure the one you choose is suitable for stripping bark.

4.   Weeding Knife

Also called hori-hori or Japanese garden knife, the weeding knife is one of the sturdiest wildcrafting tools you can rely on. You'll use this knife for digging roots, but the greatest thing about them is that they can cut through almost all kinds of clay soils. You can break up the soil and then dig up, transplant, or divide roots using the weeding knife. A Hori-hori knife is a loyal and sturdy friend that can last decades as well as throughout your foraging endeavors.

5.   Digging Fork

An alternative to your hori-hori knife, you can use a digging fork to weed the roots. A digging fork will have sturdy and square tines that can loosen soils and gently lift the branching roots out of the soil. That's why they're a better choice for digging earth than shovels or spades, as they're much less likely to damage the roots than their counterparts. You can loosen soil weed or harvest medicinal roots easily using the digging fork.

6.   Chopping Knife

Although you can rely on a weeding knife for most roots, you'll come across some tough roots that just don't budge. For those cases, it's better to have a heavy-duty chopping knife on hand to do the job.

7.   Shovel

A shovel is one of the tools you'll find stuck away in a corner in your garden shed or garage. If you don't already have one, you can get a shovel easily from any store. Once you're there, be sure to get a couple of shovels of different shapes and sizes to cover your bases. At the very least, get a long-handled one with a pointy blade, which will help break heavily compacted soil or excavate large tap-rooted plants.

8. Pruning Saw

You should always be mindful of what you break, but there will be situations when you have no choice but to prune small to medium branches and tree limbs. That's when a pruning saw will come in handy. The tools you need will all depend on your foraging plan, but a pruning saw is most handy for gathering medicinal tree bark, like black birch or wild cherry.

9. Containers

You'll definitely need a container to carry the fruits of your harvest. You'll also need a container to help you divide your portions, test your edibles, or even prepare your meals. Assorted baskets will be great when it comes to carrying or even drying your herbs, and it's easy to get these from any store. You can get any basket according to your taste, but it's better to make sure it's sturdy and safe.

Additionally, you may also need a couple of buckets to hold larger amounts of harvest, especially in the case of fruits like wild blueberry or elderberry. You'll also find them great containers for carrying muddy root harvest, and the extra water at the bottom will serve in keeping the leaves and stems fresh until you get back home. The size of the bucket depends on your needs, but three to five-gallon buckets are a good place to start.

10.   Gloves

You'll definitely need gloves to keep your hands clean from all the dirt and protected from getting spiked by stray thorns. In the worst-case scenario of coming into contact with poisonous species, or in the less perilous case of brushing through thorns or bushes, the gloves will act as the first layer of protection against danger. So, your gloves need to be thick and sturdy - think leather gloves. That said, you can keep a second thinner pair on hand for more delicate jobs. In either case, your gloves will keep your hands safe from both dirt and danger.

11.   Vegetable Brush

After you gather your roots, you'll probably need to brush off the extra soil hanging onto your precious harvest. Instead of doing everything by hand, having a sturdy and bristled vegetable brush will allow you to easily scrub the soil from the crevices and cracks.

12.   Hand Lens

A hand lens is also known as a jeweler's loupe, and there's nothing more helpful to help you ID your plants by scrutinizing their botanical parts. Your best bet is to get a 10x to 20x lens, which will give you 10 to 20 times of magnification. As you can figure out, the magnification ability of this lens is much higher than the normal magnifying lens. Most hand lenses also have integrated LED, which will make your job of spying on the flowers much easier.

13.   Fruit Picker

This will be your go-to tool for gathering fruits, especially the fruits you want to forage in the wild. Picking fruits from well-managed trees is easy, but it's a completely different story when it comes to foraging. You won't have access to a ladder, nor is it convenient to carry one - so, instead, you'll get your own fruit picking tool. The concept is simple; all you have to do is get a long-handled pole with opening claws at the end that allows you to reach greater heights and catch your fruits. You can also add a basket or a container to the pole to catch your harvest. Whether you choose to buy it from a garden center or make your own doesn't matter, as long as you have a sturdy tool.

When, How, and Where to Harvest

Generally speaking, you'll never go wrong with foraging for wild edibles during the spring. Although you may find specific species throughout different seasons, spring is usually the best time to forage for the finest greens, like dandelions, miner's lettuce, wild asparagus, and ramp. Some spring mushroom species, like morels, even rival those of the fall.

Remember that we are foraging for fun, not necessarily to keep us alive, unlike the wildlife that lives in the forests. Although we may beat our competition to the wild edibles, it's only ethical that we become conscious of the ecosystem we're disturbing.

There are a few rules that every forager must abide by. Namely, never exhaust the entire harvest of a certain fruit, and be sure to visit different places throughout your visits. Not only will doing so endanger wildlife, but it can also make you a target for endangering wild species.

Leave your foraging space neat and put back what you disturb. It's bad manners to create a big mess of dug-up earth and leave it without care.

There's isn't a specific place in which you can forage. You're free to forage for wild edibles if you come across any. However, what you should look out for are polluted lands that have been sprayed with herbicides or pesticides. The same goes for deserted cities - make sure to harvest plants that haven't been polluted by auto exhaust or other pollutants. It's also imperative to make sure the land from which you're foraging is public and not privately owned.

How to Gather Nuts

Foraging for nuts is different from gathering wild edibles. The best time to go looking for nuts is during the fall, when you're guaranteed to stumble across tremendous amounts. In most cases, the trees will drop their nuts as soon as they're ripe. Your job will be to compete with the tiny creatures who will get to the nuts first, o especially when it comes to black walnuts.

Knowing your nuts and their characteristics will save you a load of trouble down the road. Some nuts are far from tasty; others can only give you a smidgen of the edible kernel after a tiresome battle of cracking their shells. If you're looking for the easiest nuts to gather, your best bets will be green acorns or beechnuts. Both nuts can be readily eaten after harvest. You'll only need to remove the brown skin off the beechnuts first, or they are dried for storage.

Pecans and hickory nuts can also be easily picked when they ripen, as they leave their green husk and keep their shells. They're easier to crack than butternuts or walnuts, although you'll still need to use some brute force to crack their shells. Generally speaking, though, it's best to keep your nuts in their shells until it's time to eat them, whether you leave them as is or dry/roast them for a longer shelf-life.

How to Gather Fruits

The consensus is that the best time to gather fruits is when they're ripe, but the trick is knowing how to tell the difference between ripe and unripe fruits. For instance, picking fruits with a smooth exterior is a sacred rule handed down throughout the generations. While that rule may apply to a lot of fruits, like apples, pears, and cherries, you'll never taste anything as astringent and starchy as smooth persimmons. Instead, you'll savor the sweetest taste with a hint of cinnamon if you pick extra wrinkly persimmons, which indicates the fruit is ripe.

It's also important to know the proper time for harvesting your fruits. Many fruits ripen during the fall and through the winter, but some start to ripen as early as summer. Rosehips and blackberries are two examples of these fruits, and both can be eaten raw, used in making syrups, jams, and drinks, or dried and stored for cooking purposes.

Meanwhile, elderberries also ripen in the fall, but only the flowers are edible. It's also better to eat them cooked rather than raw, as they can make one sick. Be aware that they have a lot of poisonous lookalikes, although they don't produce berries like the elderberry plant. While you're watching out for plants, hawthorn berries also have poisonous lookalikes. If you do come across them, though, never eat them raw as they're terribly bitter. Instead, you can process them to be added to jams or liquors according to your desired taste.

Despite being very involved and quite a challenge at times, learning how to forage is an exciting and entertaining endeavor. With every new species you add to your basket, you get a sense of achievement that keeps you going. However, you must learn the difference between the edible plant and its poisonous lookalike, maybe even more so than learning the edible ones. Ready to keep yourself safe? Let's move on to the next chapter.

Chapter 4: Staying Safe in the Wild

In the previous chapters, we have talked about edible plants, their benefits, and how to identify them. This chapter will take some safety precautions by discussing the poisonous variety and how you can avoid them.

Not every plant is edible, and hunger can make even the most dangerous plant look delicious. Chris McCandless, the main character in the movie "Into the Wild," which is based on a book under the same name, is believed to have died after consuming large amounts of a toxic wild plant. You may think this is just a fictional story that will never happen in real life. However, "Into the Wild" is based on a true story, and its protagonist died because of a poisonous plant. So, to be safe rather than sorry, you need to be able to identify these plants and not make the same mistake.

The problem with some toxic wild plants is that they look so similar to safe edible ones. Think of it like a good twin and an evil one; they both look the same, but one of them can be very dangerous while the other is harmless. When we get hungry while we are in the wild, it is easy not to do a thorough check and confuse the poisonous plant with the safe version and trust the evil twin.

Poisonous Plants

Poison Ivy

You have probably heard the name Poison Ivy before, and no, we don't mean the Batman villain. Poison Ivy is a toxic plant that can be hard to identify because it resembles a little weed when it is still young. When Poison Ivy is more mature, it begins to resemble a furry vine, and it can be mistaken for a small tree.

The toxicity of this plant is through touch. Touching this plant will cause blisters and itchiness. The effect of Poison Ivy is so powerful that if someone chops it with a hatchet and you touch the hatchet, you will suffer from severe skin irritations. The toxin is found in the type of oil on its leaves called "urushiol," which makes the leaves the most toxic part of the plant. But, touching any part of Poison Ivy will still cause serious reactions.

You should also avoid burning Poison Ivy because inhaling its smoke can put you in the hospital. You will find this plant everywhere in the United States with two exceptions; Hawaii and Alaska. To avoid this plant, you will need to recognize it first.

Memorize this saying to help you in the future, not just with Poison Ivy but with other plants as well, "leaves of three, let it be." This means that you should avoid plants with three leaflets like Poison Ivy. However, in the South, East, and Midwest, this plant grows as a vine, while it grows as a shrub in the West and the North.

Poison Oak

The Poison Oak shares many similarities with Poison Ivy as both plants look quite similar except that the Poison Oak's leaves resemble that of an Oak tree. Like Poison Ivy, Poison Oak also contains urushiol, which causes irritation to the skin. When you touch this plant, you may not suffer a skin reaction right away. It can take hours or even days for the reaction to show on your skin. However, when it does occur, the blisters may ooze, and the rashes may turn bumpy.

Poison Oak grows everywhere in the U.S., but you will mostly find it in the West. The leaf of this plant has one side darker than the other, which is the one facing the sun, it is a darker shade of green and has tiny hairs.

Poison Sumac

Although most Sumac shrubs are quite harmless, the Poison Sumac isn't. Its leaves and berries are toxic. Like the previous plants that we have mentioned, Poison Sumac will also cause skin irritation like itchiness, and it also isn't safe to inhale its smoke if its leaves are burning. You will only find this plant in soggy and wet areas around the country. Each plant's stem has between 7 to 13 leaflets, a red stem, and light green or white berries.

In some cases, the rash caused by a Poison Sumac may show on your face or private areas, cause puss, or cover large parts of your body. If this happens to you, you must see a doctor immediately.

Giant Hogweed

Another plant you should never touch is the Giant Hogweed which belongs to the carrot family. This plant originated in Europe and is considered very harmful. The Giant Hogweed has its name for a reason, as it can grow up to 14 feet. It's quite similar to the wild carrot with its white clusters and hairy stalks, and it is very dangerous for many reasons. Firstly, your skin will become very sensitive to UV light if you touch it. If you come into contact with it and are exposed to the sun afterward, your skin will suffer from painful, dark, and deep blisters that will cause severe scarring, which can last for years.

Your skin isn't the only part of your body that will suffer if you come into contact with the Giant Hogweed, your vision will too. If you get the plant's sap in your eyes, you will be permanently blind. It is safe to say that you need to completely avoid it and if you accidentally touch it, you should wash your hands very well with water and soap and avoid the sun completely for a few days. To tell the difference between this plant and the white carrot, you will find that the Giant Hogweed has purple spots on its stems. Additionally, its leaves are different from the wild carrots.

Pokeberries

Looking at the berries of the Pokeweed plant, you could probably be tempted to pick one and eat it because they look so delicious. These berries make a tasty meal for migrating birds and animals like deer, as they don't affect them whatsoever. However, you shouldn't think they are safe just because a bird is feeding on its berries because they are highly toxic for human beings. Even in a small amount, these berries can kill a child, and a little more can actually kill a full-grown adult. No matter how delicious these berries look, you must avoid them at all costs. Identifying them is easy since they have the same clusters as grapes with brightly colored and purple-black berries. Their stalks grow up to 8 feet tall, and they are a purple-pink color.

Moonseed

The Moonseed plant is another grape look-alike that you shouldn't be tempted to try. You may believe that it's harmless because its fruits and berries resemble that of grapes, but they can be fatal if eaten. However, the one difference that will save your life is the seeds. Ripe grapes usually have 2 to 4 seeds, while the Moonseed only has one. The seeds of both fruits look different, as the grapes' ones are round or oval while the Moonseeds' look like a crescent moon, which is where its name comes from. When in doubt, or if you are unable to recognize the fruit, simply check the seeds.

Rhododendron

The Rhododendron is a Native American name that means suicide bush, so we can tell from this translation that this plant isn't safe. The Rhododendron looks like any regular shrub, and you will find it mainly in the East of the U.S. Its leaves resemble that of the bay leaves used in cooking. However, confusing both leaves can be deadly since the Rhododendron leaves are toxic. To identify this plant, brew the leaves in strong tea. If you notice a strong revolting odor, this is the toxic Rhododendron plant and should be avoided.

Holly

No one can resist berries, and Holly's red berries can tempt anyone to grab a couple to taste them. Although you may see birds feeding on this fruit, you shouldn't believe they are safe. As mentioned, some poisonous plants don't harm birds or animals but can be dangerous to us because the berries contain various toxins. Although fatalities from these berries are rare, they still happen, so caution is advised.

Horse Nettle

Horse Nettle is another delicious-looking plant that can confuse most people into consuming them but make no mistake; they are no less dangerous than any of the plants we have mentioned in this chapter. The Horse Nettle is a juicy fruit that usually has a green or yellow color and looks like a cherry tomato. You should always be careful with plants that look like tomatoes because many of the tomato's wild relatives are toxic to humans. It isn't just the fruits, but the rest of the plant also contains toxins. If you consume Horse Nettle fruits, you will suffer from abdominal pain and respiratory and circulatory systems problems. So, avoid any fruit that looks like a wild tomato when in the wild.

Virginia Creeper

Virginia Creeper grows in the north and far south of the U.S.; you will usually find them in Texas and Manitoba. Many people tend to confuse this plant with Poison Ivy, but if you take a closer look, you will notice that the Virginia Creeper has five leaflets while the Poison Ivy has three. This plant is extremely toxic and fatal.

Wisteria

You should avoid all members of the wild legume families because the non-edible and non-cultivated ones are deadly. Wisteria is a good example as it contains a substance called wisterin that can be extremely poisonous if eaten. The seeds are covered in a velvet bean pod and are flat and area dark color.

Dogwood

You will find this plant in the eastern U.S. during the early winter and fall. Like the Holly plant, Dogwood also has red berries that humans should avoid, although they are safe for birds.

Buckeye

Who would have thought nuts could be poisonous? The Buckeye trees grow in the central and eastern areas of the U.S. and are extremely toxic. The nuts are usually covered with a shiny brown shell, and the outer husk structure resembles that of the hickories. However, they are different from hickories on the inside as they are shiny brown and round, while the hickory is similar to a walnut. Additionally, the nuts of the Buckeye resemble chestnuts which can confuse some people too. The chestnuts are usually covered with needled husks, and being aware of the difference can save your life.

Bittersweet Nightshade

Bittersweet Nightshade berries are brightly colored, so if you have kids, you need to be extra careful because they may be tempted to try them. Unlike some of the plants mentioned here, the Bittersweet Nightshade is extremely toxic for both humans and animals when eaten. All parts of this plant are poisonous: the berries, sap, leaves, and bark. If consumed, it will make you vomit, tremble, and give you headaches, stomach aches, drowsiness, diarrhea, and lower your temperature. This plant grows up to six feet.

Yew Shrubs

Yew Shrubs have bright red berries, and their leaves look like a needle. The seed inside the berry is toxic to people, while the leaves are toxic to both animals and humans. Consuming these berries will stop your heart.

White Baneberry

Here is a tip that will save your life, avoid any plant with the word bane in its name because they are toxic. Baneberry is a good example. They are usually found in Canada and the eastern areas of the U.S. Its berries are white, and the stalks are red. Not only is this plant toxic, but it is also scary-looking. Although they are delicious, the berries can stop your heart and kill you instantly.

Stinging Nettle

Touching the Stinging Nettle can be dangerous because of the tiny hairs on its stems that can shoot into your skin, releasing various chemicals which can cause rashes. This plant can grow up to four and even six feet tall, and it grows in patches without branches.

Mistletoe

Mistletoe is a very popular plant usually used in Christmas decorations. It grows on shrubs and trees, and it has thick stems which are easily broken. The plant also has many branches. The Mistletoe's leaves are green and thick, while its flowers are yellow with no petals. The berries are white, small, and contain one seed and a poisonous pulp. Consuming the berries is very dangerous and causes diarrhea but can have more serious effects like slowing or even stopping your heart. This plant is also harmful to animals.

Strychnine Tree

You will find these trees in Australia, India, Asia, and Sri Lanka. The flowers of this plant have a foul smell, and the berries are in a smooth and hard shell. Consuming these berries can also be fatal.

Safety Precautions against Poisonous Plants

Now that you've learned about poisonous plants and how to identify them, you are probably wondering how to protect yourself from them in the wild. Whether you work outdoors or enjoy hiking or camping, you need to protect yourself from toxic plants. It isn't just consuming or touching these plants that can be dangerous, but you can also breathe some of the substances that they release, like the urushiol that we have mentioned earlier. This substance will penetrate your skin, nose, throat, and eyes.

To be safer rather than sorry, you will need to protect yourself - wear clothes that cover your skin so you don't come into contact with long pants, long sleeves, and high boots. We can't stress enough that every part of your body should be covered, even your hands, so you should also wear leather gloves. Wash these clothes when you get home because they may be contaminated. You should also apply a barrier cream on your exposed skin, like your face. If you are going to use any equipment like hiking poles, you should wash them thoroughly afterward. Even if you don't use the tools, but they were exposed to poisonous plants, you should still wash them with soap and water or sanitize them with rubbing alcohol.

No matter how careful we are, accidents can happen, and you may find yourself coming in contact with any of these plants. As mentioned, rashes and skin irritations usually occur when touching various plants like Poison Ivy. If this happens, you will need to isolate the infected part of your body. The rashes usually last from 10 days to 3 weeks. However, certain treatments can help speed up the process. You will also need to avoid scratching the rash so you will heal faster.

If you get a rash, the first thing you should do is to rub the infected area with alcohol or wash it with skin wash specially designed for this kind of irritation. You need to rinse the area and your hand regularly to prevent the infection from spreading.

To reduce blistering and itching, apply calamine lotion after cleaning your skin. You can also use baby powder to clean the rash, dry it, and apply a small amount of rubbing alcohol. To prevent the rash from spreading, you should wrap it in cotton gauze afterward. If there is nothing available to help you disinfect the rash, some home remedies can help. For instance, you can use vodka by applying it directly to the infected area or using a banana peel to relieve the itch.

As mentioned, the rash may spread to different parts of your body, like your eyes or genitals. You may also find yourself suffering from swelling, having trouble breathing, high temperature, and oozing blisters. In this case, you will have to seek medical help immediately. If you have tried the methods we have mentioned and see no improvements in your rashes, seek medical attention.

If you or someone you are with loses consciousness, has seizures, or difficulty breathing, they might have consumed a poisonous plant. Immediately call 911 or the emergency phone number in your area. Your mouth may also hurt or feel irritated as a result of exposure to these plants, so you should then drink water or milk.

When picking plants, you should wear gloves and don't eat any plants you don't recognize. You should also pick one type of plant at a time; you don't want to mix different types together and risk contaminating your safe edible plants. If you eat a plant and find the taste strange or unpleasant, stop eating immediately.

Be careful of white berries because many of them are toxic. If you see an animal or a bird eating a plant, you shouldn't assume it is harmless. Additionally, plants consist of different parts, so if a part is safe, it doesn't mean that the rest of it is. Some people also think that cooking a toxic plant will make it safe; this is a misconception. A toxic plant remains poisonous even when cooked. As mentioned, smoke from burning toxic plants is also extremely dangerous so never burn them or any plant you don't recognize. Follow these tips whenever you are in areas where poisonous plants usually grow to protect yourself, including your pets. You should also familiarize yourself with all of the toxic plants on this list and the safe edible ones mentioned in previous chapters to be safe in the wild. When in doubt or unable to identify a plant, avoid it completely.

Chapter 5: Fundamentals of Foraging

In order to be able to make use of edible wild plants safely, not only do you need to know about the plants and which kinds of plants are safe to eat, but you also need to know about foraging. In itself, foraging is a complete skillset that takes time to master. Whichever type of resource you are foraging for, you need to know how to go about your search in an efficient way to actually find the right resource. This involves both bits of knowledge of the plant you are after and the skill to know how to find it.

This becomes increasingly important as you start looking for more difficult to find plants, and also when you are looking for plants that can easily be confused with poisonous look-alikes.

In this chapter, we will cover all the basic things you need to know about foraging. However, it will take time and practice to perfect this skill set.

The Edible Plant Test

If you find yourself in a situation where you can't spot anything you can accurately identify as being edible, there is a way for you to gauge the safety of a plant before you eat it. This will help you eat a plant out in the wild without risking your life.

1.   Smell – If the plant smells foul and unpleasant, it's best not to eat it. While it may smell bad due to its condition, it could also be an indication of other dangerous chemicals.

2.   Touch – If it passes the smell test, touch the plant to the inner side of your elbow and hold it there for a few minutes, then remove it. Wait for 15-30 minutes to check if the area starts to itch, redden, burn or feel irritated in any way. If it passes this step, then proceed.

3.   Kiss – Press the plant against your lips and wait to check for any reactions. Wait at least 15 minutes, and if your lips still feel fine, then you can proceed to taste.

4.   Taste – Take a small bite of the plant, chew and hold it in your mouth without swallowing. Keep in mind that most plants will taste quite unusual, especially if you have never eaten a raw plant before. However, it should not taste extremely bitter, spicy, or unpleasant. It will have a general earthy taste, and if it is extremely unpleasant, spit it out.

5.   Eating – Before you actually eat the plant, wait at least a few hours after the taste test to see if your mouth has any reactions to the juices that came out of the plant. Wait a minimum of

four hours before you take a bite and swallow. When you do decide to eat it, only eat the parts that you have tested, such as the leaves or the seeds. Eat the plant in very small quantities, just a bite or two at first. Then allow it four to six hours to go through your digestive system and check for any reactions. If you feel any kind of dizziness, nausea, digestive problems, or anything else, then don't eat any more. If everything goes fine, then you can eat a slightly bigger bite the next time. Keep increasing the amount while checking for effects, and build up the quantities that you consume.

This is a very time-consuming process, but it's the only way you can ensure that a plant will not kill you. Once you have identified a plant to be safe, you can continue using this in the long term, so it's well worth your while to invest the time in analyzing whether or not a plant is safe to eat.

Basic Foraging Rules

The rules that you apply and the criterion through which you select plants to forage will be heavily dependent on the environment that you are in, as well as the specific plant that you are looking for. As a rule of thumb, there are a few basic rules that you can use which will help you stay safe in situations where you don't know what to do.

1.   Animals – Don't rely on animals to find your food. While this is the approach that a lot of people have used in the past and is one of the ways through which we have diagnosed which plants are safe to eat, this is not always the case. Some plants can only be digested by other animals, and while they seem to be perfectly fine for them, they can be fatal for humans, even in small quantities. If they aren't fatal, they can make you extremely sick, so it's best not to eat what animals are eating as you don't know how well it will work for you.

2.   Child Safety – If you're foraging just for fun during a picnic or while you are out camping, keep an eye on your children and make sure they are very clear about the fact that they are not free to eat whatever they want. Children, being the inquisitive beings that they are, often don't understand the significance of studying what they are eating. Foraging is just a fun activity in which they can eat random things in the jungle. Make sure they don't start experimenting with things on their own, and make it a policy for them to first show you something that they think is safe to eat before they eat it. Even small amounts of the wrong plants can be very dangerous for a child.

3.   Use Smell – In many cases, you will find a plant that looks like something that should be fine to eat, though it's not. One of the best things to do is to check the scent of the plant and see if it has any bad odor to it. Smelling the plant on its own may not be enough. Try to break off a leaf, crush it up and smell that. Some plants are completely odorless, but when you crush a leaf and smell it, you will realize that it does not smell food friendly.

4.   Urban Plants – Ideally, you should not be foraging in urban areas, and even if you are, make sure it's not at a private property or an area that receives a regular flow of road traffic. Plants in urban environments and even those located near roads always run the risk of being polluted with chemicals in the form of pesticides and pollutants. If you do have to eat a plant that is found in such an area, it's best to cook it or at least give it a very thorough wash.

5.   Prepare – Some wild plants are meant to be cooked before use, and not all wild plants are safe to eat right out of the ground. Similarly, some plants cannot be eaten whole, and you should know which parts of the plant you can eat. Make sure you prepare the plant before you eat it.

6.   Go Slow – You may have come across an area that has a lot of different plants which all look safe to eat, and you may be tempted to try them all. Don't. Some plants have a reaction only several hours after consumption, and even though they are safe to eat, you never know if you will have a reaction to a plant, or which plant is the cause of your problem. Ideally, you should only try one per day so you can see any effects up to 24 hours after you have eaten it.

7.   Need – When foraging for food and wild plants, it's very important to keep track of how much you are taking from the environment. Sometimes you will come across a resource that you need in abundance, and you will be tempted to get as much as you want. But wild plants and fruit both rot easily and can't be stored for very long. It's much more sustainable to take as much as you need and then come back later when you need more. The great thing about plants is that they won't run away. Mark that spot, and you have a mine of natural resources that you can use whenever you need to.

Tools

If you are foraging plants and other edible greens, it's a good idea to have a knife or a pocket multi-tool that can help you cut different plants and easily slice certain parts of an edible plant. While you can get by with your hands for most plants, it's better not to have the plant fluid on your hands. It can be especially difficult to get certain types of plant fluid off your hands, given the fact that water can be hard to find out in the wild. You don't want to have to use up all your water on washing your hands.

Moreover, certain plants, such as cacti, will require a tool if you want to eat them. You will have to remove the spines, which can't be done with your bare hands. Some plants which may look like they can easily be handled actually have microscopic hairs on both the stems and the leaves, which can be dangerous to handle with your bare hands. The toxicity of plants varies a lot, and while some may just prick you a little or irritate your skin a bit, others can have much more serious consequences, not to mention that if you are handling sensitive plants such as fungi, it is a lot easier to cut a portion off rather than trying to break it with your hands and ruin the entire plant. In other cases, you may find it much easier to cut out a fruit or slice a vegetable off the entire plant rather than having to break it or rip it off.

Having a tool also makes foraging much safer for the environment; clean cuts and precise slices cause a lot less damage to a plant and help it to continue to grow so that you can use it again later in the future. Handling certain plants can ruin the entire plant making your foraging efforts harmful to the environment. Also, for certain things like nuts and seeds, you will need at least a knife to be able to process them further. Quite often, you will need to cut through thick protective layers to reach the edible part of a plant, and having a tool to help you do this not only makes it easier but also makes it possible.

Where to Forage

As a beginner, your best option is to start In urban environments that have well-documented plant growth and a limited diversity of available plants. Be sure you stay away from private property and other locations where it is not permissible to forage.

Usually, in urban environments such as your backyard or local parks, you will find plants that are more easily identifiable and closely related to known edible plants. Due to the presence of a lot of other common plants such as vegetables and fruit, the chances of you coming across something that is edible is much higher through pollination and the fact that there are orchards and farming areas close by. A lot of plants that are growing nearby for human consumption get scattered around the city and are commonly available.

If you are looking for certain plants that only grow in specific conditions, you will need to know what kind of environment they grow in to find them. Truffles, for example, are extremely difficult to find. While there is an equal likelihood that you will find them in both urban and wild environments, the fact that they are mostly found underground makes it challenging to locate them. However, if you know which signs you should be looking out for on the surface and plants that they grow near, you should be able to find them.

When foraging in the urban environment, you need to be extra careful about eating plants right away. Even in places that look like they have been left unattended for quite a while, you never know when they were last sprayed with chemicals and what kinds of chemicals were used. Moreover, plants in cities and busy areas collect a lot more pollutants from the natural environment. While they help clean the air and may look healthy, you never know what kind of substances are deposited on them. Even if you are foraging out in your backyard, you need to be very particular about washing and cleaning plants before eating them, or better still, cook them before you eat them. Things such as manure and compost can be very dangerous if ingested, so be sure to properly treat your wild plants before you eat them.

Common fruits are also very easily available in urban areas, but you need to make sure that they are not someone's private property before you forage them. If in doubt, it's always better to ask someone. People will be much happier allowing you to take some of their fruit when you ask rather than just picking it without their permission. As you get more experienced, you can start to venture out to more remote areas where you will find a larger variety of plants, and you will also have access to plants that are native to certain kinds of environments.

When to Forage

The kinds of plants, fruit, and natural resources that you find in an area will vary a lot through different times of the year. Some plants that flower in the winter will not even be present in the summer, and vice versa.

Here is a small breakdown of what you can expect to find at different times of the year.

January – For most places around the world, January is wintertime, and this is the season when fruit, berries, and nuts can be found in abundance. Fruit such as blackberries, whitebeam berries, crab apples, and hawthorn berries can be easily found. While these fruits are great on their own when they are fresh, January is when you can make a lot of jams from this fresh produce to use throughout the year. These fresh berries can be preserved in a variety of ways, so get creative and make the most of this fantastic month.

Other resources you will find during this time include nuts and seeds. You can harvest acorns, hazelnuts, walnuts, and chestnuts. There are also several seeds that you can harvest year-round, but they are especially plentiful in the winter. Moreover, these nuts and seeds can be ground into flour and used for a myriad of purposes.

March – This is usually the onset of spring, and it is the time of year when you will be able to find a lot of smaller, more tender plants that you can eat as they are or incorporate into different cuisines. Some of the most commonly found plants during this season are yarrow, hairy bitter cress and meadowsweet. Depending on where you are, you may find many other wild plants that are native to that region. Most of these plants are loaded with minerals and vitamins and make for very hearty and healthy meals. While these can be difficult to store, it's best to make use of them while they last.

May – As the summer comes close to its peak, a lot of small plants and even larger fruit trees are coming into season. Plant activity is at an all-time high during this season as the conditions are favorable for a wide variety of plants. For foragers, this is the time to look out for things such as chickweed, hawthorn, mallow, and red clover. The great thing about these plants, and this time of the year, is that you will find many of these in your backyard. If you don't see these exact plants, you will find a lot of other vegetative growth in and around your garden that is completely edible. So, you won't have to go far to find something to eat, though if you do venture out, this is when you will find a huge diversity of plant life. Most of these small plants are best eaten raw, as part of a salad or as a garnish to a meal, but you can also combine them to use in cooked meals. Sorrel, for example, is a great green that you can commonly find in urban areas and is very similar to spinach, and can be used in both hot and cold dishes. With its tangy leaves and succulent stems, it's a refreshing addition to any kind of dish.

July – This is close to the peak and even a little after the peak of summertime for many places around the world. While there are several types of small plants that are still available, you will also be able to find a large number of fruit trees in full swing in this season. Some of the interesting plants that you can look into during this time of year include chanterelle, chickweed, wild strawberry, and bilberry. This is the second season in which you will have access to a lot of fruit that can be stored. Wild strawberry makes for an especially potent jam and, while it's much smaller than store-bought strawberries, it is extremely pungent and packed with a lot of nutrients. Unlike the store-bought variety, the greener strawberries of the wild strawberry plant can be extremely sour and even inedible for some people, so make sure you get the nice red ones. Being a very sensitive fruit, they are easily spoiled, so you may have to look around before you get a few in good shape. You can also find a lot of fruit during this season that you can enjoy fresh and also preserve for the rest of the year.

September – Autumn time is when hedges and trees come into full swing and offer their benefits in the form of nuts and seeds. A lot of fruit is also going to be available along with many kinds of plants. Some of the best things to gather during this season include beech nuts, rosehip, wild raspberry, and sloes. Sloes are particularly good during this time of the year, especially after the first frost as their skins soften, and the juices become more concentrated. You can use these berries to make the famous sloe gin which is a fantastic drink for the cooler evenings of wintertime. These sweet, tangy jewels also make a fantastic jam, and the fruit can be used to make sloe vinegar.

Chapter 6: Safety Measures in the Wild

While there are a variety of plants to be found in the wild, not all wild plants are edible. Some wild plants contain toxins that can be harmful to humans and animals. Poisonous plants can cause skin irritation, rashes, and some can even pose a serious risk to life. Out of all poisoning cases, plant poisoning contributes to almost 10% of them. If you have a homegrown garden, poisonous plants can find a way to grow in the shadows. It is vital to identify and eliminate any wild poisonous plants growing in your backyard. It can pose a serious risk to small children and pets.

The toxins in a poisonous plant are capable of causing sickness and can lead to death if consumed or ingested. In some cases, coming in contact with a poisonous plant is enough to cause serious damage. Also known as secondary compounds, the toxins present in some wild plants are the waste products of the chemicals present in the basic metabolism process. These chemicals may include oxalates, toxalbumins, glycosides, saponins, and alkaloids. These toxins are harmful to animals, humans, and vertebrates in various ways. While some effects are subtle such as birthing defects and reduced weight gain, other responses can be fatal.

For millions of years, the toxins and chemical substances in wild plants have evolved to fend off herbivorous insects. If an animal has a weak immune system, the chances are high that the animal will get poisoned if it comes into contact with these poisonous plants. Some of the toxic substances found in wild plants can alter after entering an animal's body and cause serious damage. For example, cyanogenic glycosides lead to the production of cyanides within the body. It can cause the animal to have violent spasms and can result in a painful death.

While researchers are continuously trying to find out about new toxins from wild plants, it is essential to beware of some of the most commonly found poisonous plants. In this highly descriptive chapter, you will discover the various ways to identify a poisonous plant. In addition to this, you'll also discover some rules to avoid these dangerous plants and keep yourself away from harm.

How to Identify Poisonous Plants

When it comes to identifying plants that are poisonous for living beings, one description does not fit all. The factors to identify a poisonous plant may vary greatly depending on the plant species, environment, and other aspects. Some old sayings like "leaves of three, let it be" may apply to certain plants like poison oak and poison ivy but are not sufficient as a tool to identify other poisonous plants. In addition to this, various non-poisonous plants look similar to common poisonous plants. To identify and differentiate poisonous plants from harmless lookalikes, you should be well-versed in the properties and characteristics of the most common poisonous plants found in the wild.

Poison Oak

With striking similarities to the leaves of an oak tree, the leaves of a poison oak look a lot like its cousins, poison ivy and poison sumac. The sides of a poison oak's leaves that face the sun are of a darker shade of green as compared to the other side that generally faces the ground. In addition to this, the sun-facing side of the poison oak's leaves has tiny hair growing on it. Commonly found in western countries, poison oak is a shrub with leaves of three, just like poison ivy. However, pacific poison oak may appear to be like vines. Poison oaks can be identified by their green or yellow flowers as well as their white or greenish-yellow berries clustered on the shrub. With that said, coming into contact with the plant sap can result in rashes and oozing blisters. It may take some time for your skin to react to urushiol, the plant sap.

Poison Ivy

Easily recognized by the oily sap on its leaves, poison ivy is closely related to poison oak and poison sumac. While poison ivy usually grows as a vine, it may grow as a shrub in the north. It is identified by its green or yellow flowers along with a cluster of amber or greenish-yellow berries. Poison ivy typically has tiny hair on its leaves, and three leaves are budding from the same stem. Poison ivy is easily noticeable in the wild due to its vine structure and three leaflets. However, the poison ivy found in the western regions does not take the shape of a vine but rather looks like a low shrub. If your skin comes in contact with poison ivy, you may have an allergic reaction that causes your skin to itch, swell, and turn red.

Poison Sumac

Usually found in swamps and wetlands, the poison sumac can be identified as a woody shrub that has at least 7 to 13 leaves arranged in pairs. If you find clusters of green berries drooping from a woody shrub, the chances are high that you have come across poison sumac. Another characteristic that can help you identify poison sumac is its cream, pale-yellow, or glossy berries. If your skin is exposed to poison sumac, you can develop a rash and may feel very itchy. With that said, inhaling the smoke of burning poison sumac can also be dangerous. If the rash covers more than 25% of your body and you notice pus coming out of the rash, immediately consult a doctor. In addition, Taking a cool shower and applying calamine lotion on the rash will help you reduce the itching. However, it may take you a week or more to completely recover.

Poison Hemlock

Native to Europe and South Africa, this plant is an invasive weed that can grow in a wide variety of environments. The seeds and roots of poison hemlock are the most toxic. Poison hemlock can grow as big as 8 feet tall. The roots of poison hemlock penetrate deep into the ground, and the plant has an unpleasant odor. The stem of poison hemlock may have dark maroon or purple spots. It can also be identified by its distinctive and separated leaves that have a striking resemblance to a large parsley plant. If this plant is eaten or ingested by animals or humans, it can poison them. In addition to this, when your skin comes in contact with the poison hemlock's oils, you can fall sick.

Stinging Nettle

This plant is popular for its stinging leaves. The stem and leaves of stinging nettle are covered with tiny hairs, also known as trichomes. One of the best ways to identify a stinging nettle is to look for the stinging trichomes on the stems of the plant. In addition to this, the stems of stinging nettle have no branches in some patches. The plant can grow up to 4-7 feet tall. With that said, the tiny hairs on the leaves and stems of stinging nettle have round tips that break off when touched. The trichomes contain various chemicals like histamine, serotonin, acetylcholine, and formic acid. These chemicals can cause painful skin irritation, allergic reaction, and severe itching if the trichomes pierce the skin. The effect of the stinging hairs can last up to 12 hours. In addition to this, if a person or an animal's skin is pierced by a massive number of trichomes, it can poison them and possibly be fatal.

Bitter Nightshade

Found in a wide variety of habitats, the bitter nightshade is an invasive perennial weed that can grow throughout the year. This plant is known to reach a height of up to 6 feet wherever it finds suitable support. Bitter nightshade has star-shaped purple or yellow flowers that resemble an arrowhead. In addition to this, the fruit of the bitter nightshade is a red and juicy berry that looks like a tiny tomato. While it is edible for some birds, it can be poisonous to animals and humans. However, the attractiveness of soft and juicy berries can draw children to consume them. Eating the fruit of bitter nightshade can cause diarrhea, drowsiness, headache, stomach ache, and vomiting. If consumed in large quantities, it can be poisonous and may require immediate medical attention.

Giant Hogweed

Usually found near streams, farms, and ditches, the giant hogweed requires rich and fertile soil to thrive. This plant can be recognized by its small white umbrella-shaped flowers that have ingrained creases on them. In addition to this, the stems of this plant are hairy and have purple patches on them. The giant hogweed can grow as gigantic as 15 feet tall. With that said, coming in contact with the sap of giant hogweed can be dangerous. The sap of this plant is known to be phototoxic.

If you come in contact with the sap of the giant hogweed plant, it can prevent your skin from protecting itself from the sun. If the area of contact is large, you may experience severe inflammation on your skin. In addition to this, it may lead to serious skin problems like phytophotodermatitis. You may also experience burns, blisters, or scars as your skin grows more sensitive to ultraviolet rays. It is crucial to protect your eyes from the sap off the giant hogweed plant because it can impair your vision permanently. With that said, the reaction may start as early as 10 minutes after the sap comes in contact with the skin. The symptoms can last for several days.

Foxglove

Popular for its looks, the foxglove plant is grown in many gardens throughout the world. It has bell-shaped flowers that can be pink, purple, white, or yellow. While the seedy fruits of a foxglove plant are as attractive as their flowers, they are poisonous, just like all parts of the flowers. The foxglove plants contain a lot of chemicals that can slow down or disrupt the heart. Deadly glycosides present in the foxglove plant can be poisonous for livestock and humans. This is why the foxglove plant has plenty of sinister names, such as witch's gloves and dead man's bells.

Consumption of the foxglove plant can dangerously intoxicate humans. The symptoms of ingestion of the foxglove plant may include nausea, diarrhea, headache, abdominal pain, vomiting, and crazy hallucinations. In addition to this, the victim may also suffer from cerebral disturbances, jaundice, irregular heartbeat, slow pulse, and visual impairment. With that said, people also report loss of appetite, weakness, drooling, seizures, and dilated pupils. In extreme cases, an overdose of the foxglove plant may also result in death.

Jimsonweed

Recognized by its strong odor, the jimsonweed plant is an herb that can grow up to 4 feet tall.

The leaves of this nightshade plant are about 3-inches long, and the flowers are shaped like trumpets. With that said, jimsonweed is a toxic and poisonous plant. The nectar from the white flowers of the jimsonweed plant can make you thirsty and nauseous. In addition to this, the seeds and leaves of these plants can make you feel feverish, increase your heartbeat, and reduce your pulse. Consuming this plant or inhaling the smoke from it can cause loss of memory and hallucinations. In addition to this, the toxic effects may also include seizures, fever, dry mouth, impaired vision, vomiting, and breathing problems. If a human consumes 15 to 25 g of jimsonweed seeds or 15 to 100 g of its leaves, it can poison the person and also result in death.

Oleander

One of the most poisonous shrubs found in the wild, the oleander plant is recognized by its long leaves that have a velvety finish and that usually grow in groups of three. Another notable feature of the oleander plant is its flowers that grow at the end of the branches. The bright colored clusters of flowers on an oleander plant can vary in color from pink, red, and white. However, every part of this colorful plant is poisonous. Even a single oleander leaf can kill an adult or animal. This dangerous shrub contains toxic components that can cause breathing problems, bloody diarrhea, vomiting, abdominal pain, excess saliva, directed pupils, and irregularities in pulse. In addition to this, if your skin has prolonged contact with an oleander plant, you may suffer from skin irritation and inflammation. Since the oleander plant has a very bitter taste, humans and most animals refrain from consuming it. This is why the risk to lives due to the consumption of the oleander plant is low.

Rules to Avoid Poisonous Plants

When you are out in the wild, you encounter a lot of dangers. Poisonous plants alone pose a great risk. If your skin comes in contact with a toxic plant, you may suffer from skin rashes, irritation, and even inflammation. If you consume a poisonous shrub, you may experience headaches, vomiting, nausea, and breathlessness. Getting poisoned by a plant is one of the worst things that can happen. In addition to this, the probability of coming across a poisonous plant is extreme. So, what can you do to avoid the risk to life? In this section, we'll discuss the various rules you can follow to avoid dangerous plants.

Learn to Identify

The first step to safety is to be informed about the various poisonous plants. If you're aware of the nature and type of the plants, the threat is automatically reduced. However, you should always be aware of your surroundings when you're out in the wild. Quite often, people unknowingly scrape their hands or legs against a poisonous plant while hiking through a thick patch. The symptoms may take some time to show up. All you can do is hope that it's not too late. With that said, it is wise to carry an illustrious field guide with you that includes information and images of all types of plants and wildlife. In addition to this, you can learn in advance about the most common poisonous plants found locally in the area you're traveling to. It will not only help you protect yourself from potentially dangerous plants but also give you something to talk about with your companions in the wild.

Be Prepared for the Wild

One of the best ways to avoid poisonous plants in the wild is to be prepared for the worst. As a rule of thumb, always cover your body whenever you go out in the wilderness. Long pants, full sleeves, and proper hiking shoes can help you avoid your limbs being exposed to dangerous plants.

However, if the heat is unbearable and you decide to wear shorts, make sure to compensate by pulling up your socks as high as you can. This will help you protect your legs from being exposed to poisonous plants. In addition to dressing properly, you can carry a bottle of outdoor skin cleanser in your backpack. If you are exposed to a poisonous plant, you can rub this cleanser on your skin to reduce any itching or rashes. If you don't have an outdoor skin cleanser with you, you can wash the exposed area of your body with cool water and gently clean it with a cloth.

Watch What You Eat

Out in the world, you may feel tempted to pluck a juicy red fruit from a plant nearby. That may not be the wisest of choices. When you are out trekking or hiking, do not touch, pick, or eat an unknown plant. Since poisonous plants tend to thrive in wild settings, your chances of coming across a harmful weed are high. By eating an unknown plant, you will be putting your life at risk. Be it berries, nuts, seeds, leaves, or stems; you must always be cautious of what you eat in the wild. In addition to this, it is potentially dangerous to make tea from an unfamiliar plant or suck nectar from its flowers. It is also crucial to remember that some poisonous plants look similar to edible plants. If you are in doubt, it is best to avoid it completely. Do not be tempted to eat fruits or berries or anything else that you come across in the wild unless you're completely sure.

Wash Up

If you've hiked through a large part of the wilderness, it is essential for your well-being to set aside your gear and clothes to be washed as soon as you get a chance. Your clothes may be carrying toxic substances if you brushed up against a poisonous plant. Separating your hiking clothes from your clean clothes will help you limit exposure to poisonous substances. In addition to this, always make a point of washing and cleaning yourself if you've been around wild plants. With that said, some people love taking their pets on treks and hikes. While animals are as prone as humans to poisonous plants, they can carry and spread the poison much faster.

If you too love taking your pet as a companion on your trips, remember to give your pet a nice clean bath with soap and water after your trip.

To conclude this illustrious chapter, let us take a brief look at the key takeaways. Out in the wild, the chances of getting exposed to poisonous plants are high. From rashes and skin irritation to dehydration and vomiting, poisonous plants can have very adverse effects on your health. While there are some similarities between poisonous plants, it is difficult to clearly define their characteristics. The best way to identify poisonous plants in the wild is to learn about them, look at their pictures, and study the potential symptoms.

The most commonly found poisonous plants include poison ivy, poison oak, poison sumac, poison hemlock, stinging nettles, bitter nightshade, giant hogweed, foxglove, jimsonweed, and oleander. Each plant has its distinct identity and symptoms. While the dangers in the wild are many, you can easily avoid exposing yourself to poisonous plants by following some simple rules. Always make sure you dress appropriately, be aware of your surroundings, learn to identify poisonous plants, be prepared for the worst, avoid eating wild plants, carry a bottle of outdoor skin cleanser, and wash your things after spending time around wild plants. If you suffer from serious rashes or other symptoms, seek medical attention immediately. Being informed and applying these safety measures in the wild can help you stay safe from most dangers.

Chapter 7: Preserving Wild Edible Plants

The wonderful thing about wild edible plants is that they can provide you with a lot of nutrition. This nutrition comes at almost no cost, and if you eat a diet composed of these wild plants, you'll be able to get more nutrients than you get with your regular store-bought diet. However, the main issue with wild plants is availability.

When you harvest the wild plants, they immediately start degenerating, and if you don't preserve them soon enough, you'll not be able to use them for long. Most of these wild edible plants grow edible parts only during the summer, and if you live in an area where the winter's harsh, you'll have a very short window to preserve your food. You have to understand the proper preservation techniques if you want to store these edibles for later use.

Another thing that you should keep in mind is that the storage technique has to be right, or else the food that you store may rot or develop harmful fungus. There are a variety of preservation techniques that you can employ to preserve these foods in a safe manner. We'll be looking at all the different preservation methods that you can use to store the edible plants for future use without any chances of spoiling them.

We'll also be looking at how these stored foods can be transported so as to maintain their freshness and to ensure that no losses occur. You may need to travel from one place to another, and it can lead to unnecessary spoilage. You may not have access to a refrigerator or preservatives, which can increase the odds of your food getting spoiled. The section on transportation will explain the proper transportation methods and the precautions you should take.

Even though you might have tried your best to preserve these edible foods, some of them will inevitably go bad. It's just an important aspect of storing these plants that can't be avoided. However, you should know when these plants have gone bad so that you don't consume anything that may be injurious to your health. We'll be discussing in brief how you can spot any edibles that have gone bad to the point of no return. This way, you can learn how to avoid any health hazards and only consume the edible plants that are still consumable.

Preservation Methods

There are a variety of preservation methods that can be used that do not require much high-tech equipment to keep your plants consumable for a long time. Whichever one you choose will depend on the different pros and cons of each method.

Make sure that you properly clean all the wild harvest that you have collected. Properly rinse it after soaking it for a while. Soaking is a very important step as it can help you clean off any dirt or debris from your wild edibles, and it can also help to reinvigorate the greens and keep them fresh. The wild plants stored this way will be tastier and more fresh when you start preserving them.

While some methods are fairly low-tech and easy to do, other methods may require a bit more effort on your end. So, let's find out methods you can use to enjoy the fruits or plants of your harvest for a long time.

Drying

The age-old method of drying out the plants to remove moisture is one of the most efficient methods of preservation. Even when using this method, you can go for the top-notch options by utilizing electric dehydrators, or you can use some ingenious solutions to do it cheaply. The electric dehydrators can eliminate almost all of the moisture from your food, but they don't come cheap and can get very expensive.

Another option that you can opt for is a solar drying box. These boxes will save you a lot of electricity and will be cheaper in the long run but will cost you a lot initially. However, these solar drying boxes can be built at home if you're even a little experienced in building things yourself. Building one yourself will save you a large chunk of money that you'd otherwise spend on buying a factory-made unit.

Another way that you can dry out your edible plants is to use the natural energy of the sun. This is a free option that'll do its job nicely, considering the price you pay for it. Just try to keep your edible plants out in the sun until they don't change their color anymore. Once the color has changed, you can remove them from the sunlight, and it'll last you for a pretty long time. To expedite this process faster, you can try to slice the edible plant into smaller pieces and apply a little lemon juice before you place it under the sunlight. This will ensure that the edibles dry out faster and don't attract any microbes.

Most of the dried-out weeds and herbs can be ground into powdered forms, and that'll help you keep away any moisture by packing it in an airtight container. Anytime you need to use these materials, you can simply rehydrate them or blend them with oil to be used as dressings or chutneys.

This method works out great with almost all fruit and vegetables. If you have a fleshier vegetable or fruit, you can sprinkle a bit of salt on it, and it'll result in much better dehydration. You'll find the best results when drying out leafy vegetables with more surface area, and the fruit will remain leathery even after they dry out.

Pickling

Another great method to preserve your wild edibles is to pickle them in a brine of salt or vinegar. You can go with either of those options depending on the flavor and aroma you desire. It's a very simple and effective way to preserve vegetables because of the ample availability of both these ingredients. Just try to do it in a very sterile environment for the best results. If you fail to eliminate any unwanted bacteria from your containers or water, it'll result in a pickle that tastes weird and smells funny.

If you go through the entire process correctly, you'll achieve preservation that enhances the taste of the bland food and is very beneficial to your health. You'll need to keep your pickle refrigerated for its longevity, and when properly kept, it can last as long as 6 weeks. A good pickle will keep your gut populated with good bacteria, and you'll also be able to digest the foods better.

Many people choose to add additional ingredients like garlic, ginger, clove, or dried chili peppers. These additions provide your pickle with a complex taste that will increase the variety of your palette. You can preserve almost any wild plant like chickweed leaves, plantain, or dandelions this way, and it'll most likely still taste good.

Blanching and Freezing

Blanching is a very simple process in which you have to put your vegetables in scalding water or under steam for a short period. This has many benefits for your health because it cleans the surface and kills any microorganisms that may be on the vegetable skin. The other very useful benefits are the enhancement in color, the slowed down loss of vitamins and minerals, and the softening of the vegetable, which makes it easier to store.

After you're done blanching, all you need to do is put the food in the freezer. Once the food is frozen, you can pack all of it into plastic bags that can be used very conveniently. You can just take out a packet whenever you need it and thaw it before using the vegetables for cooking. It's highly advised that you don't re-freeze your food once you thaw it as it can lead to a loss of the quality of your vegetables.

Even though frozen food can't be used in a salad, it can definitely be used to cook other nutritious food. Refrigeration technology has become so cheap and effective compared with any limited source of energy like solar energy. It's a time-tested method for preserving vegetables and is your best bet if you want to preserve your vegetables' taste and quality for a long time.

You can preserve your vegetables for a long time, unlike with the other methods, which can barely last a month to a season. Frozen veggies are fresh up to 8 to 10 months after being packed, and that's plenty of time for you to grow a new harvest. Try to refrigerate your vegetables as much as you can because this way is rather easy and longer-lasting.

Some Things to Keep in Mind

Before you embark on your journey to self-sustainability with a basket in your hand, there are a few key things you should keep in mind. Be doubly sure that the weeds that you're collecting don't have any sort of pesticide or herbicide sprayed on them; consuming these weeds could result in severe medical issues and are to be avoided at all costs. Even plants that grow near the road will most likely be contaminated by heavy traffic and other toxic pollutants, so avoid these as well.

You should also ask for permission before you collect plants from anybody's private land. It's not a good idea to trespass, and you should avoid it at all costs, especially if the gun laws where you live are lenient. If you ask the owners beforehand, it'll be much safer for you, and you can gather all the required plants without any worry.

Another thing that you might need to watch out for is if a plant is poisonous or not. Don't even think about taste testing an unknown plant, as it can lead to a catastrophic scenario where you might get seriously poisoned by the plant. Always take someone experienced with you and try to keep learning about the edible weeds in your area. After a while, you'll have a good knowledge of what to pick and what to avoid. Keep a reference picture handy if you don't know what you're looking for, and you'll be able to spot the edible wild plants much more accurately.

Other precautions are more general in nature, but nonetheless, more important. You should try to maintain proper hygiene by properly cleaning and washing the collected greens since you don't know if a dog may have peed on it in the past. Also, try to avoid wild vegetables and foods if you have some serious allergies. If your allergy flares up after eating an entire meal, you'll have a severe shock that can be life-threatening.

Transporting Wild Edible Plants

Procuring and preserving wild edible plants is all fine until you're forced to transport them. You have to be conscious of the pace at which you transport your edibles because that will influence the condition in which it arrives. It might seem like a simple task from the outside, but it actually takes a lot of effort to achieve the desired results.

If you want to ensure that your preserved edibles don't get spoiled, then it's a good idea to clean up the transportation space. If you can't keep the surroundings clean, then it may lead to contamination 0f your preserved foods, and that will eventually lead to spoilage of the entire crop. Cleaning your transportation is one of the most straightforward ways to ensure safer transportation and can be easily completed in less than an hour.

Another important aspect that you have to keep in mind is the temperature at which you store your wild edible plants. All the different wild edible plants require different temperatures to be stored, and you have to keep this consideration in mind. It's also very important to maintain and constantly regulate the temperature so as to ensure that there is no deterioration of the quality of edibles. You can purchase a refrigerator or hire a refrigerated truck that will give you the best cooling options. If you choose to purchase a mini-fridge or cool box, it'll be an investment that will be well worth it in the future.

The shelf life of the preserved edible plants is another factor that should be kept in mind while transporting. If you can't keep the preserved edibles refrigerated, then it becomes more important to consider the shelf life of each product. The shelf life of different plants can vary by a huge margin, and you have to know each and every plant's durability to better transport them to remote locations. Fresher edibles will always be better than a plant that has wilted away. Fresh plants will retain more of their nutrients over a longer period of time, when compared to edibles that have been out in the open without any preservation.

Another thing that you should keep in mind is the seasonality of the wild plants that you harvest. If you can transport the plants in the harvest season, then you'll have much better results because the plants will be fresher. Different plants have different seasons of growing as well, and if you're well-acquainted with the entire schedule, then you'll be able to harvest, preserve, and transport them more efficiently.

The little mistakes like improper packaging can be a huge issue as well. If you don't stuff enough packaging material into your shipment, it'll lead to breakage of the containers, which will lead to huge losses. Also, make sure you package your containers tightly and seal them the right way so that you don't face any unexpected leakage. If you can avoid these basic mistakes, you'll be able to save a lot of money that would've otherwise been wasted. The advice that safety is better than cure applies perfectly in this situation.

You may face many issues along the way that you didn't even expect. However, if you're prepared well in advance, then you'll be able to avoid the associated risks. The issues that may pop up later on can be delays, spillage, spoilage, and much more. If you can take proper precautions before transporting the preserved plants, then you can avoid a lot of unnecessary trouble later on.

Identifying Spoiled Edibles

A rotten or spoilt plant can cause so many issues that it can cripple you for days on end. You have to be careful while eating these edibles because if you don't examine what you eat first, you'll be suffering from intense gastrointestinal issues or even death. The ability to identify when a wild edible has gone bad will come in very handy. You'll be able to identify if something has gone bad while harvesting it or even after the preservation is completed. You can't preserve anything indefinitely, which is why knowing when something will expire is a very crucial skill to develop.

The very first thing that almost everyone does to identify if something has gone bad is to smell it. You can pretty easily identify if something edible has gone bad by comparing its previous smell to the way it currently smells. If you feel like the odor has turned strong and unpleasant, you should probably discard the product, as it may get progressively worse.

You can also test a sample for toxicity by placing a small sample of it on your skin. If you exhibit any symptoms like rashes, itching, burning, numbness, or swelling, then you'll need to discard the product immediately. However, if you're still unsure about the toxicity of the product, then you can try to swallow a little bit of it and wait for a few hours. After waiting for some time, if your body has still not exhibited any symptoms, then you can proceed to consume the item safely. However, if you suffer from any issues like vomiting, diarrhea, or stomach aches, then the preserved plant may be poisonous, and you should safely discard it somewhere no animals can access it.

It's also important to know the causes behind these spoiled foods as it'll help you avoid any unnecessary spoilage in the future. The main culprits like moisture, fungus, light, high temperature, microbial growth and more can spoil the preserved items rather quickly. The age-old way of preserving anything has been to put the preparation in a cool and dark place. This cool and dark environment is best for these items because there is less of a chance of them getting spoiled by light and warmth.

The other wild edible plants that haven't been dried or are in an intact form will be of higher nutritional value by removing as much moisture as you can. The foods we eat contain a lot of moisture, and the presence of this moisture causes all the proceeding rot and decay. If you can control and maintain this moisture at the right levels, your food will stay fresh much longer.

This chapter was a brief introduction to preserving wild edible plants after they've been properly harvested. We saw a lot of benefits of the different preservation techniques utilized by different people. You now have a proper beginner's guide to the amazing world of wild plants. You can always refer back to this chapter for tips and methods when preserving something at your home.

We also explained how you can spot the food that is about to go stale or has already been infested by harmful bacteria. There are certain cues to look out for and once you learn these cues, you'll be an expert at identifying the food that's consumable and the food that's not. We even covered how to transport your preserved wild plants and prevent any accidental damage like spilling or leaking. You learned all the different methods one can employ for taking your goods from one destination to another while still maintaining the amazing quality of your preserved goods.

Chapter 8: Edible Plants in Your Backyard

If you are thinking of converting your backyard into a thriving food-producing garden, you should know the type of plants to grow. Not every plant can give you the expected yield in a small garden. Therefore, you need to select the edible plants carefully and take other necessary measures to ensure that your backyard garden is a success. This chapter outlines tips and tricks on how to start cultivating your edible plant garden.

Plan Your Garden

Like any other business, you need to plan your garden properly before you spend money on anything. You must take time to assess the amount of space that you have in your backyard that you can convert into a garden. Having a big space in your backyard does not necessarily mean that you can turn it into a successful garden. You should start small and experiment with different plants to see how they perform before you expand your garden.

To grow edible plants in your garden, you must choose a place with the best light from the sun. Many garden plants require exposure to sunlight for about six to eight hours every day. This means that you must carefully study your yard and choose the best location for your garden. Make sure that the position you choose has easy access to water. The other thing you should know is that some edible plants can grow well in places with partial shade. When choosing edible plants for the garden, make sure you have information about their requirements to grow well.

When planning your garden, you must also define its purpose so that you choose the right plants. You need to determine the type and amount of food that you would like to grow in your backyard space. The type of edible plants that you grow in your garden is a matter of personal preference. All you need to do is ensure that you pick the right crops that are easy to grow. Some garden crops take longer to ripen, whereas others will be ready in about 60 to 90 days. You should do your homework first before you buy plants for your garden. Remember that other plants like pumpkins, melons, and corn require a large space to spread out, and they also take time to ripen.

A garden requires attention, so make sure that you have enough time to tend your plants. You can start with a single raised bed and closely monitor to see how things go. You may be surprised that a small space can produce plenty of food. From there, you can consider expanding your garden if you are happy about the initial results. You must prioritize the quality of the crops you grow, rather than quantity.

Check the Quality of Soil

Soil is probably the most important component that will determine the health and success of your garden. The first thing you should do is get a sample of soil from your garden to test for acidity or alkalinity. You can buy a pH kit from a hardware or nursery in your local city. The appropriate soil pH that you need for your garden should be neutral to a level of slight acidic (pH 6 to 7). If you have acid soil around your home, you can adjust its composition by adding calcium in the form of lime or dolomite.

You need to do some research to gain insight into how acidic soil affects plant growth. It is believed that alkaline soils are not easy to correct, but the addition of compost and sulfur over time can help improve the soil. Composting is good for your garden since it is purely organic. You also need to understand how soil alkalinity can impact plant growth. Soil that is rich in organic material is ideal for any type of plant. Organic nutrients are free from harmful chemicals that can damage the soil and produce poor-quality crops. Quality soil should have organisms like earthworms that enhance the decomposition process of organic matter.

You must also ensure that your garden has good drainage, and the soil can retain nutrients and moisture. Issues like water pooling in certain areas indicates poor drainage. Waterlogging severely affects plants since it indicates that the soil is too compact, and it cannot absorb water. The other cause of poor drainage can be attributed to poor landscape design. You need to ensure that the landscape in your garden consists of a good drainage slope.

The other challenge with soils is that some have faster drainage rates. For instance, sandy soils have an equally fast drainage rate and may require constant watering during hot days. You can improve this anomaly by adding organic matter like manure and compost to the soil. Apart from buying cheap stuff from hardware stores, you can build a rich compost for your garden at home. Compost is good for your garden since it provides the nutrients required by the plants, and it is also cost-effective.

Choose Easy-to-Grow Crops

When you understand the soil type at your home, you can choose the ideal plants to grow. Some crops like watermelons, broccoli, and giant leeks can look gorgeous in the garden, but you should not be tempted to grow them when you are just beginning your garden. Instead, you should focus on tried and tested plants that are easy to grow and productive. For instance, crops like radishes, peas, kale, salad greens, mint, tomatoes, chives, and zucchini are perfect choices that you can consider.

Make sure you plant your favorite foods that you enjoy eating instead of wasting your time and space. You can consult your local seed company to get an idea about the best plant varieties that suit your regional climate. Some plants are easy to grow, and they are highly productive. If you are a beginner, you need to choose your favorite vegetables, fruit, and herbs together with other edible plants that you love to eat.

It is a good idea to grow crops that you like to see in your garden. You may need other plants in large quantities, whereas you may not need a lot of herbs. You will not need to buy garden produce like tomatoes from the supermarket when you have a thriving garden at your home. Vegetables and flowers can also grow well in your garden. The good thing about growing flowers is that you can use them in salads, and they also add a good flavor to raw dishes. There are other plants like fruit, herbs, and vegetables that you can eat raw.

Another vital aspect that you must consider when choosing edible plants relates to seasonality. Some plants are productive throughout the entire year, whereas other crops do well in certain seasons. You can read the information about different plants on seed packets. It is essential to consult the stall at your local nursery to get an idea about the ideal plants that you need to get for your garden.

Some plants require a lot of water, while others can survive with little water. Too much water can lead to the rotting of the roots, which ultimately leads to unprecedented losses. All types of edible fruit trees like apples, lemons, and apricots require little attention once they begin producing fruit.

Choose Between Seedlings or Plant Seeds

You can buy seedlings from a nursery in your local area, and the main advantage is that they are ready to plant in your garden. The seedlings are usually grown by experts, and they are tested for quality assurance before they are sold to the customers. When you buy seedlings, you can choose the exact crops that you want, and this will make the gardening process easier.

However, you can save money by growing vegetables from plant seeds. You can learn a lot of new things and grow a variety of crops if you nurse your seeds. If you plant edible crops from seeds, you can increase variety in your garden. The problem with overreliance on seedlings is that the local nursery shops may not have the plants that you want for your garden.

You can purchase edible plant seeds online if you cannot get the ones that you want locally. Once you get a collection of different types of seeds, you can start your home nursery, which can help you generate money from the sale of seedlings. It is vital to build a greenhouse if you are concerned about productivity in your garden.

Invest in the Right Garden Tools

You need to invest in the right tools to prepare your edible plant garden in your backyard. A backyard garden is usually small, but you will need several tools. It is vital to focus only on the basic tools that you require for your small plot so that you do not waste a lot of money. The following are the basic garden tools and accessories you must have.

• Gloves- Gardening can turn out to be a thorny issue if you handle everything without proper gloves. When choosing your gloves, make sure they are not too bulky since this can lead to poor performance. Poorly fitting gloves can lead to accidents or other elements like blisters. Get gloves that are water-resistant if you want to improve your gardening experience.

• Pruning Shears- You need to get a pair of hand pruners to help shape the plants that are growing out of control in your garden. The pruners come in different shapes and sizes. For a small garden, you need to get something easy to handle in your palm.

• Garden Fork- A garden fork is a must-have tool that you can use for digging and turning the soil to mix manure. You can also use a fork to mix a compost pile. If you are working with dense soil, this tool is very effective since it consists of sharp prongs that can penetrate any type of soil.

• Hand Trowel- You need this handy tool to perform activities like transplanting plants and taking out weeds from vegetable beds. You must get a tool with a comfortable handle.

• Spade- You need a spade to move mounds of soil to different places in your garden. You can also use this important tool to dig holes in your garden for planting new crops.

• Rake- Helps you clean up leaves and other debris in your garden. Rakes come in different styles and sizes. Some are adjustable, and these are convenient since you can use them in different settings.

• Garden Hose- Water is a critical component that determines your garden's life. You should get a hose with an adjustable nozzle to ensure that you can control water pressure, so it does not damage your plants. A watering wand also gives your plants a gentle shower-like watering system. This irrigation system is designed to ensure that water steadily seeps into the ground.

• Wheelbarrow- Comes in handy if you want to move soil, compost, or any other heavy material around your garden. A wheelbarrow makes life easy in your garden since it is easy to use and maintain.

It is important to get the right storage space for these tools to maintain a thriving garden.

Choose the Right Planting Method

Another important consideration that you must make concerning your edible crops is the way that you should plant them. Traditionally, many people used to plant vegetables in low rows. Others would just plant crops randomly without following any specific pattern. You need to create raised beds for your vegetables, and they are advantageous in that they provide clear access to the plants in your garden. There are footpaths in between the raised beds, which makes it easier to manage your garden.

With raised beds, you can significantly reduce the amount of weeding required. The wonderful aspect about a raised bed is that it promotes the fast growth of plants. You can also enhance productivity with a raised bed which is normally packed with compost and other components that provide nutrients to the crops. Raised beds also play a pivotal role in keeping your food organic which is good for your health and your family. Scrap that is usually disposed of in landfills can also be used to make raised beds. Reusing this material can benefit plants in several ways.

The other benefit of using raised beds is that you can use a planting method that helps you to divide the crops using a grid. With this technique, you can grow more crops in a little space.

However, you need to take note of the spacing requirements for different plants in your garden. You must leave sufficient gaps between the plants so that they get enough space to grow. You also need to keep your garden neat to help you identify the issues that may need attention.

Control the Weeds

Weeds can be a menace in your garden since they can grow even in the best plots that you can imagine. Weeds will grow as long as conditions promote plant growth, like sunlight, moisture, and nutrients in the soil. However, the main challenge is that natural weeds grow faster than edible plants. Grass will ultimately impact the growth of crops in your garden. There are different measures that you can take to fight these unwelcome visitors in your garden.

You can consider chemical options to clear weeds in your garden if you are concerned about improved productivity. Commercial herbicides are designed to kill grass which helps to promote the growth of crops. However, you need to choose the right herbicide since they come in different forms. The other problem with using herbicides is that they can impact the soil and the environment. Artificial chemicals can also affect the quality of plants and your health in the long run. Enlightened gardeners are now seeking other alternatives in their quest to promote green farming.

If you plant your crops on raised garden beds, you will realize that you experience fewer weeds. You should also pull the weeds by hand, and this is the safest option of eliminating these undesired components in your garden. If you get rid of the weeds using physical methods, you will preserve soil and plant health over a longer period. You should not wait for the grass to grow too big since it can affect the growth of your plants.

Label Your Crops

You must keep your garden organized by labeling the crops. This stage may seem insignificant, but it can make a big difference. When you plant something, use a plant marker and include details like type of crop and planting date. This helps prevent the confusion of sowing seeds in the same place twice before they start to germinate. Plant markers also give you an idea of the date when you should expect to begin harvesting the crop. Some plants take longer to ripen than others.

You must treat your garden with an open mind and accept failure. In some cases, other crops can fail, and this is perfectly normal. Therefore, you should not get frustrated or lose hope. You must do some research and learn from your mistakes to try to identify the cause of the problems you encounter so that you can avoid them the next cropping season. You should remember that a successful gardener spends a lot of time learning from their mistakes. You also need to open up to new techniques and treat gardening as a hobby.

Tips to Maintain Your Edible Garden

To maintain a successful edible backyard garden, you must first plant suitable crops that are favorable to the climatic conditions prevailing in your area. Some plants require sunlight for optimum growth, while others can thrive in cooler temperatures. You should ensure that you select your favorite crops to avoid wasting the limited space available in your garden.

You must remove the weeds regularly from your garden since they can end up competing for soil nutrients with your crops. This will affect the growth of edible plants in the garden. Compost all the weeds that you remove from the vegetable beds to produce nutrients required by plants to grow. All fruit scraps and vegetable materials should be shredded before composting. Organic manure is good for the growth of healthy plants that are free from any artificial chemicals. The problem with artificial fertilizers is that they can affect the quality of soil in the long run.

Another important consideration that you should take into account is using mulch to conserve moisture in the soil. You can add mulch and other garden material to your vegetable beds to ensure that the moisture does not quickly evaporate. Mulch can also save you money in terms of reduced water bills depending on the area where you live. You must rotate the plants in your garden regularly. You can change the crops once each season or every year to preserve the soil nutrients. Crop rotation can also go a long way toward helping reduce the outbreak of diseases.

Pests can be problematic in your garden, but you need to find safe methods of addressing the problem. For instance, you can apply non-chemical remedies like chili and garlic spray to scare away the pests without killing them. Some insects play a crucial role in promoting pollination, which leads to the development of fruit.

Gardening is an exciting hobby that provides you with edible plants of your choice. If you want to grow some edible crops in your backyard garden, there are different steps that you should take.

You need to plan your garden and site it in a good location with access to direct sunlight and close to a water source. It is vital to check the quality of soil and choose suitable crops that can give you better yields.

Chapter 9: Edible Wild Plant Recipes

It can be difficult in some instances to determine whether a wild plant can be eaten or not. In some instances, like coming across a mushroom you're uncertain about, definitely avoid it. Just because an animal is consuming a plant doesn't mean it's safe to be eaten by humans.

Here are the wild plants that can be used safely and incorporated into cooking.

Burdock

Burdock can be spotted by its obvious burrs. If the burrs aren't present, then see if the plant has a rosette of oval, pointy leaves without a stem that grows close to the ground in its first year. The leaves of the burdock plant are edible. However, if the plant is older, the leaves can be quite tough and taste better when they're cooked. If the feet are young, they can be eaten as well as the flower stalks. Burdock has an earthy taste, with sweet undertones. This plant resembles cocklebur, whose leaves have to be cooked in order to get rid of the toxic elements.

Burdock roots can be cooked and consumed fairly easily. The root of this plant is very popular in Asia and works great in dishes like soups or braises. The root can be peeled, sliced, or even eaten raw. When eaten like this, it looks like radish and has an artichoke-like flavor.

It will oxidize fairly quickly, so once it has been cut, it should be placed into lemon water to prevent it from turning brown. One way to enjoy this delicious wild plant is to roast it. If you keep the skin on, you can enjoy the nutty taste it has to offer. If you aren't a fan, you can peel the skin. If the skin is kept on, ensure you wash the roots super well to get rid of any dirt. You can then slice them up, work quickly to prevent them from oxidizing. The oxidation does not affect the taste or nutrients but it looks a lot better when it isn't oxidized.

Add the sliced burdock root into a bowl with a dash of olive oil, salt, and pepper. Spread them onto an oven tray and roast at 400F for around 15 minutes. Once the roots have turned golden, flip and let them roast for around 10 minutes. Roasted in this way, the root tastes delicious and nutty. If you want to go the extra mile, you can add a dash of sour sauce and sesame seeds.

Kinpira Gobo - Burdock Root Stir Fry

Ingredients

- 1 burdock root

- 2 carrots (peeled)

- 1 tsp white sesame seeds

- 1 tsp dashi powder

- 180 ml water

- 2 tbsp soy sauce

- 2 tbsp sake

- 2 tbsp kirin

- 1 tbsp sesame oil

Method

1.   Mix the dashi powder and water in a bowl, add the soy, mirin and sake, and stir. This is the sauce.

2.   Wash the burdock root, and slice into small strips. Soak the strips in water to keep them fresh. Before cooking, drain the water and wipe off any excess water. Slice the carrots into strips.

3.   Heat the oil in a pan on medium-high heat, add the burdock and carrot strips, and stir-fry these for 3-4 minutes.

4.   Add half of the sauce and keep stir-frying. Once the liquid appears to evaporate, pour in the

rest of the sauce. Turn the heat down and simmer until the sauce has thickened.

5.   Top with sesame seeds and serve.

Dandelions

The amazing thing about these wildflowers is that every part of the flower is edible. When the flower is young, it's best to eat the leaves raw, although cooking does remove some of the bitter taste. Dandelions are a bitter-tasting plant in general, although this has benefits according to Traditional Chinese Medicine. The roots of dandelions can also be eaten. Usually, they are consumed when they are dried and have been ground. Some even consume this as a substitute for coffee and this is where the bitter taste comes in handy.

Dandelion Root Coffee

1.   Start with a bunch of dandelion roots. Wash them thoroughly.

2.   Slice them up.

3.   Arrange them on a dehydrator and allow them to dry for about an hour.

4.   Chop the dried roots up.

5.   Place them in an oven and roast them for half an hour at 200ºF. They need to be dark brown and dried all the way through.

6.   Let cool, and then grind the roots down. Roast them again for about 5 minutes at 180ºF.

7.   Use around 6 tbsp of the grounded roots with 500ml of boiling hot water and leave for half an hour.

8.   Strain this into a pan and then reheat it whenever you want to enjoy your delicious dandelion coffee.

9.   You can serve this with milk and honey if your tastebuds desire.

Dandelion Pumpkin Seed Pesto

Ingredients

•   ¾ cup pumpkin seeds

•   ¼ cup grated parmesan

•   3 garlic cloves

•   2 cups dandelion greens

•   ½ cup olive oil

•   1 tbsp. lemon juice

- ½ teaspoon salt

- black pepper

Method

1.   Preheat the oven to 350ºF. Roast the pumpkin seeds until fragrant, roughly 5 minutes. Once done, take out of the oven and cool.

2.   Add the garlic and pumpkin seeds to a food processor and chop into fine pieces.

3.   Add the cheese, dandelions, and lemon juice and process until everything is combined. You may need to stop occasionally to scrape down the sides. It might be quite thick and hard to process, so give it a while.

4.   Add the oil and process until the pesto is a smooth paste. Add your salt and pepper.

Dandelion Greens with Garlic

Ingredients

- 2 cups of dandelion greens

- 2 tsp salt

- ¼ cup oil

- 1 clove garlic

- ½ cup onion

- 1 small chili

- black pepper

- parmesan cheese

Method

1. Get rid of the roots of the dandelions.

2. Add water to a bowl along with 1 tsp of salt. Drown the leaves in the water for around 10 minutes, then remove and rinse.

3. Cut the leaves until they're about 2 inches.

4. Bring the leaves to a boil in a pan along with the rest of the salt; leave them to cook for about 10 minutes. Ensure the pan is uncovered.

5. While the dandelions are cooking, heat up the oil and sauté the onions, garlic, and chili.

6. Strain the leaves and add them to the onion pan.

7. Season to taste.

8. Top with parmesan cheese and serve.

Dandelion Green and Potato Salad

Ingredients

- 2 cups of potatoes

- large bunch of dandelion greens

- 3 tbsp olive oil

- 2 garlic cloves

- 1 head of chicory

- 1 can white kidney beans

- zest and juice of a lemon

- 2 tbsp ricotta

- salt and pepper

Method

1.   Boil the potatoes, drain and slice in half.

2.   While the potatoes are boiling, trim the dandelions and chicory. Rinse and cut into large pieces.

3.   Heat up the olive oil, add the garlic and stir until it turns golden.

4.   Add the greens and sauté for around 2-3 minutes.

5.   Season with salt and pepper.

6.   Add the kidney beans and the potatoes to the pan. Mix everything together and add the zest, lemon juice, and ricotta.

7.   Toss everything, so everything is evenly coated.

8.   Check the seasoning and add salt and pepper if necessary.

This salad can be enjoyed warm or chilled.

Wild Garlic

In Europe and Asia, this plant is abundant during the springtime. This plant can be added to a salad to make wild garlic pesto or soup. The plant is easily identified and can be consumed raw or cooked. Wild garlic is related to the garlic that you're used to. Native to Britain, this plant signifies the beginning of spring. Until fairly recently, it was a secret favorite of foragers, but it has now become less popular.

Wild garlic tends to grow on the edge of damp woods, usually close to streams or brooks. In some places, you may find that a large amount is growing, with an entire area covered in wild garlic.

It smells strongly of garlic and onion and can easily be identified through its strong scent. The bulb of the plant can be used as a small onion, the shoots can be used in leaves or as herbs. The big leaves can be chopped up and eaten either raw or cooked. You may treat them similar to spinach leaves.

Avoid picking wild garlic that has a lot of white flowers as this points to the plant being older, which usually means it tastes a little woody or bitter. Ensure you remove soil from the wild garlic and wash it in cold water. When cooked, the flavor becomes a lot less potent. Just like spinach, this plant wilts, so you may need to cook a lot to get the amount you need. If you find that the taste is quite strong, you can mix the leaves with spinach.

One way to preserve wild garlic is through making wild garlic butter.

Butter is an easy and delicious way to add flavor to dishes as the fat is great at carrying flavor. Because wild garlic is only around for a short while, preserving it helps elongate how long its delicious flavor can be used in food. Butter can be stored in a freezer for months without going bad or losing taste.

If you have a ton of wild garlic that you want to preserve, whip up a batch of wild garlic butter. It can be used to season vegetables, add to your Sunday roast or add a big knob on top of your steak.

Wild Garlic Butter

Ingredients

- ⅔ cup of unsalted butter

- ¼ cup of wild garlic leaves

- 1 tsp sea salt

Method

1. Ensure the leaves are washed and dried and chop finely. A sharp knife should be used to ensure that the flavor is preserved.

2. Add this to the butter along with the salt. Mix well. Taste, and add more salt if needed. The butter is now ready to be used.

3. If you want to freeze the butter, the best way is to wrap it is in cling film.

4. Open up your sheet of cling film, then wipe it to smooth it out. Do this again so you have 2 layers of film.

5. Then begin spooning out the butter into a log shape in the center of the bottom quarter.

6.   Lift it from the bottom and begin wrapping it around the butter tightly. It should resemble a baton shape.

7.   Keep rolling until the cling film is wrapped very tightly around the butter log. Tie knots at both ends, ensuring the air has been squeezed out.

8.   Cut off excess film at the ends and pop it in the freezer.

9.   If you need to use the butter, take it out 10 minutes prior, then slice it into a coin-like shape. The rest of the butter can be returned to the freezer. Remove the cling film from the butter circles and use it however you desire.

Wild Garlic Pasta Dough

This pasta has a wonderful green color and the delicious taste of wild garlic. This recipe contains no salt, so when cooking your pasta, ensure you add salt to the cooking water. Because the dough is so flavorful, you can't keep the sauces pretty simple. The recipe calls for 00 flour which is an Italian milled flour that is used for making pasta. If you don't have any on hand, you can substitute it with unbleached plain flour.

Ingredients

- 20gm wild garlic

- 1 egg

- 1 egg yolk

- 150gm 00 flour

Method

1.   Finely chop, wash, and fry the wild garlic.

2.   Add the egg, egg yolk, and wild garlic to a food processor and blend until combined. You can also mix by hand.

3.   Add the 00 flour and mix or blend until the dough turns into breadcrumbs.

4.   Knead until it turns into dough for about 10 minutes. Keep kneading, so the dough becomes strong and flexible. This helps give your pasta a nice bite and is an important part of the method. The dough may be hard to work with initially, but it will become easier as you keep kneading.

5.   Eventually, the dough will become smooth and have a pale green color with bits of wild garlic. Cover the dough in cling film and leave it for an hour.

6. After an hour, roll out the dough. You should be able to roll it and cut it into strips or use a pasta machine.

7. Add the pasta to salted boiling water and cook for around 2 minutes.

8. Drain, and your pasta is now ready.

Conclusion

Since time immemorial, the history of humanity is strongly tied to its ability to adapt to the environment and closely interact with nature for survival. Wild edible plants have played a pivotal role in the survival of humanity through different adaptation stages. The early hunter-gatherers relied entirely on edible wild plants for food and medication. Wild edible plants consist of parts that can be consumed and used to heal naturally. These edible plants have nutritional value, and they provide nutrients like fibers, vitamins, fatty acids, and minerals.

With time, people in different geographical regions have since adopted a variety of edible plants to become part of their staple diet. For instance, plants that used to grow naturally are now cultivated in different places, including backyard gardens in many homes. These plants are specifically meant for domestic consumption. Typically, almost all commercial plants that we see in various farms and gardens originated from wild plants. Some of the plants have since been modified genetically to produce the current crops we grow in our gardens.

This book highlighted different tips and tricks that can be used by beginners to identify, plant, harvest, and prepare some of the best edible plants in their backyard gardens. Gardening is an exciting hobby that offers food and many health benefits to different people. If you want to grow an edible garden, you should consider the type of plants that you will grow, like seeds, herbs, flowers, berries, and any other plants that you can consume.

Edible plants provide a lot of benefits compared to pharmaceuticals and other processed foods. However, to learn the effectiveness of wild plants, you should have the skill to identify the different plants used. The major issue here is that not all plants are edible, since others are poisonous. Consuming poisonous plants can be dangerous since it leads to loss of life in some instances. Therefore, you should make sure that the plants you grow in your plot are safe for human consumption.

With the right edible plants in your garden, there are several benefits that you can gain. Wild edible plants boast quality medicinal value that can help you and your family enjoy good health. In today's age, some people not only grow edible plants for domestic consumption but also sell surplus produce to other people. If you are not going to sell any surplus, you should know how to store your edible plants for future consumption.

Drying edible plants is a traditional method that has been commonly used since the early days of the discovery of these plants. You should store dried edibles in a dry and cool place away from moisture and direct sunlight. If stored properly, the dried plants can have an average shelf life of about two years. If you want to grow edible plants in your garden, it is imperative to know the types of crops that you will plant. Edible plants come in different forms, and you should know that they do not always give you the same yield. You also need to plan your garden successfully to ensure that it is a resounding success.

When planning your garden, make sure that it is located in a place with access to direct sunlight. Apart from planting food-producing crops, you must also consider other plants that can be used for medicinal purposes. For centuries, different types of herbs have been used to cure minor illnesses and even life-threatening diseases. During the contemporary period, different modern medicines are extracted from roots. Drugs made from natural herbs have fewer side effects which makes them excellent medicines.

Whether planting your own garden or foraging in the woods, you can always enjoy the amazing and healing benefits of wild edible plants

www.ingramcontent.com/pod-product-compliance
Lightning Source LLC
Chambersburg PA
CBHW060325030426

42336CB00011B/1212